Practicing While Human

A Doctor's Journey Beyond the White Coat

Ryan Nadelson, MD

AAPL

Print 978-1-960762-55-9
Ebook 978-1-960762-56-6
Published by **American Association for Physician Leadership, Inc.**
PO Box 96503 | BMB 97493 | Washington, DC 20090-6503

Website: www.physicianleaders.org

13 8 7 6 5 4 3 2 1
Copyedited, typeset, indexed, and printed in the United States of America

PUBLISHER
Nancy Collins

PRODUCTION MANAGER
Jennifer Weiss

DESIGN & LAYOUT
Carter Publishing Studio

COPYEDITOR
Patricia George

To Farah, who keeps me steady.

To Cannon, Cyra, and Camille,
who keep me grounded.

To my mom and dad, my brothers and
sister, and to my in-laws, whose love has
shaped both my life and my work.

ACKNOWLEDGMENTS

This book began not with permission, but with persistence. I wasn't handed an opportunity to write; I simply began, without a roadmap or guarantees. Along the way, rejection came often — from outlets, journals, and gatekeepers alike. But instead of closing the door, each rejection became fuel. What could have been a reason to stop became the reason to continue.

To my wife, Farah: You carried the unseen weight of this journey. Your steadiness kept me balanced when the demands of medicine and writing could have tilted me off course. Your patience, strength, and unwavering belief in me made room for this book to exist. This is as much yours as it is mine.

To Cannon, Cyra, and Camille: You remind me daily that perseverance is not abstract, but a lived practice. Resilience is built one choice at a time: to get up, to try again, to believe in yourself when the world doesn't. You are my grounding and my constant inspiration.

To my parents and family: You gave me resilience long before I needed to test it. The roots you planted gave me stability to weather storms, and the wings you encouraged gave me the courage to keep moving forward.

To my patients: Thank you for entrusting me with your stories, your vulnerabilities, and your lives. You have been my most enduring teachers in humanity. Every exam room conversation has reminded me that medicine is not about perfection, but about presence.

To my mentors from Northeastern to the American University of Antigua to Mercer: Thank you for shaping more than my clinical knowledge. You modeled perspective, humility, and persistence when I needed it most.

To my colleagues and close friends at the Northside Hospital Diagnostic Clinic: Thank you for standing by me through the daily rocky road of medicine. Your support kept my head above water when the weight of the work threatened to pull me under. You've walked beside me not only as teammates, but as friends.

To Nancy Collins and the AAPL team: Thank you for believing in the value of physician stories and carrying this one forward with care.

To Kevin Pho: Thank you for opening the first door, for amplifying my voice, and for reminding me that the physician narrative still matters.

To the physicians who have had the courage to use their voices: Thank you. To those who have shared their stories for years, who have inspired others to pursue medicine, and who have overcome enormous odds to arrive at their calling — you paved the way. Your example made it easier for me, and for countless others, to believe our voices matter too.

And finally, to you — the reader: Writing is born of solitude, but meaning is born of connection. If there's one thread running through these pages, it's this: Rejection is not an ending; it is a beginning. May these reflections remind you that perseverance is never reserved for the extraordinary — it is built, one decision at a time, by the refusal to quit.

TABLE OF CONTENTS

AUTHOR'S NOTE

A YEAR AGO, IF YOU HAD TOLD ME I would be signing a publishing contract, I would have laughed. Writing a book was not part of my plan. I was a physician, a husband, and a father of three — my days already full. Whatever energy remained went toward getting through them, not imagining something more.

But sometimes life does not announce itself with ambition; it arrives quietly, as a tension you can no longer ignore. And when it does, you are left with a choice: Step toward what is asking for your attention or look away.

This book did not begin as a book. It began as a need.

There were things happening in exam rooms that did not belong in progress notes or quality metrics — moments of doubt, moral weight, quiet resilience, and meaning that lingered long after the visit ended. I carried them home. They stayed with me. Eventually, I needed somewhere to put them.

I found that space unexpectedly, through a small online community of physicians writing honestly about their work and their lives. For the first time, I realized there might be room for people like me — doctors without formal writing training or literary credentials, but with experiences that demanded expression. I wrote a short reflection and shared it publicly.

It was not polished. It was not strategic. It was simply true.

People read it. Some recognized themselves. That surprised me. More importantly, it clarified something I had not fully understood before: Honesty, when offered without pretense, still carries weight. I kept writing.

Those early pieces led to broader conversations — places where colleagues, leaders, and patients might encounter the same questions I was wrestling with. One essay became another. Then another. Each time, I tried to name what so many of us in medicine feel but rarely articulate: the tension between competence and doubt, endurance and erosion, presence and burnout.

Over time, a pattern emerged. These were not isolated reflections; they were connected — threads circling identity, purpose, and what it means to practice medicine while remaining human. What I had been writing in fragments began to feel like chapters.

That realization changed everything. The manuscript grew slowly and imperfectly. Essays were rearranged, expanded, discarded. Some no longer fit; others demanded more space. New pieces emerged to fill gaps I had not known existed. There was no blueprint — only a persistent sense that the story was unfinished.

Eventually, it became clear that this was no longer a collection of essays; it was a book.

I knew the odds. First-time authors without formal literary credentials rarely land traditional publishing contracts. Still, I sent the manuscript out. I waited. Silence stretched doubt thin. Rejections arrived — polite, efficient, final.

I remember opening one of them in the parking lot of my children's school, watching parents walk past with coffee cups and backpacks while I sat there wondering if this was the moment to let go. But something quieter and steadier answered back: Keep going — not because success was guaranteed, but because the work felt necessary.

Through a chain of generosity and chance, the manuscript eventually reached an editor willing to read it not as a long shot, but as a voice attuned to this moment in medicine. When the contract arrived, I read it twice. There was no résumé behind it. No roadmap. Just the work.

This book was not born from a master plan. It grew the way medicine itself often does: unexpectedly, in the margins of life, when you are paying attention but not trying to control the outcome.

It is not proof of writing ability; it is proof that persistence matters, that honesty still resonates, that stories shaped in exam rooms and quiet moments can find their place.

After signing the contract, I returned to the very first piece I had shared online. It was short, raw, and unpolished — a doctor trying to put words around experiences that did not belong in a chart. At the time, it felt small. Now, it feels like the beginning.

Beginnings rarely announce themselves. They arrive quietly, disguised as something insignificant, waiting only for us to take them seriously.

PREFACE

This is not just a book about medicine — it is a book about being human in a world that demands certainty when it rarely exists. Medicine is my lens, but the questions explored here are not confined to exam rooms or hospital corridors. They are the questions many of us carry in quiet moments: What do we do with doubt? How do we endure when the path ahead feels unclear? What sustains us when certainty slips through our fingers?

Beneath the white coat and the steady click of the keyboard lies the same struggle faced at kitchen tables and in classrooms everywhere: the tension between doubt and resilience, the longing for connection, the restless search for meaning. The practice of medicine sharpened these questions for me, but it never offered simple answers. Instead, it taught me something more enduring: Uncertainty is not a weakness to be overcome, but a condition of being human.

If you have ever questioned your path, carried a burden in silence, or longed for presence in a world that too often shouts over stillness, this book is for you. These pages do not offer prescriptions; they offer stories — moments of failure and persistence, heartbreak and grace — that shaped me as a doctor, a father, a partner, and a human being.

They are reminders that the qualities we are often taught to suppress — vulnerability, courage, compassion — are the very qualities that life, and medicine, most demand.

In these pages you will not find certainty. You will find the courage to stand in its absence. Because whether in the clinic, the classroom, or at the kitchen table, the question remains the same: How do we carry on when certainty slips away?

Perhaps the answer lies not in mastering the unknown, but in choosing to show up anyway — with presence, honesty, and heart.

PART I

Becoming the Doctor

This is where the journey begins — not with knowledge, but with identity. Doubt collides with resilience, and the question becomes: Will I find my place in the white coat? I've come to see that the white coat was never meant to erase my doubt, but to carry it, to teach me that moving forward, even with uncertainty, is its own kind of strength.

AT ITS HEART, MEDICINE is less about certainty and more about connection, resilience, and presence.

Before I could write about what it means to be a doctor, I first had to become one. And that journey began not in the neat arc of a textbook or the prestige of a lecture hall, but in the messier terrain of doubt, sacrifice, and the quiet resilience that forms when no one is watching.

The early years of medicine are rarely heroic. They are, instead, marked by fluorescent-lit nights and questions that echo louder than answers. I remember walking hospital hallways that seemed to stretch forever, the smell of antiseptic in the air, the squeak of nurses' shoes against the tile, the sting of stale coffee keeping me upright. I remember wondering — more times than I can count — if I truly belonged.

For a long time, the white coat felt like an ill-fitting costume. It hung heavy on my shoulders, as though it belonged to someone else — someone surer, sharper, more destined for the role than I was. And yet, each morning, I put it back on — not out of confidence, but out of necessity. I told myself that maybe, if I wore it long enough, I would grow into it.

That is the paradox of becoming a doctor: You are asked to shoulder the weight of authority while still learning how to hold yourself up. On paper, I was making progress — passing exams, moving through rotations, collecting the credentials that mark the path forward. But inside, a quiet, persistent sense of inadequacy trailed me everywhere.

It showed up when I compared myself to classmates who seemed effortlessly brilliant. It showed up when I stumbled through my first patient presentations, my voice cracking as I searched for the right words. It showed up when I realized that the lives of real people — messy, fragile, unpredictable — were far more complex than anything the textbooks had prepared me for.

And yet, amid that inadequacy, something else began to take root. Resilience does not arrive as a thunderclap; it grows slowly, almost imperceptibly, in the act of showing up again and again. Each time I slipped and stood back up, each time I admitted I didn't know and chose to learn anyway, each time I returned to the bedside despite the weight of self-doubt — those were the moments that shaped me far more than any exam ever could.

Looking back now, I see those years less as a test of knowledge and more as a test of becoming. Medicine was asking not just what I knew, but who I was willing to be when certainty failed me. The journey was never about perfection — it was about presence. It was about discovering, piece by piece, that the white coat did not define me. What defined me was the courage to step into it, even when it felt too big.

These first chapters of my life as a doctor are not about arrival. They are about beginning, about learning to live with inadequacy, to wrestle with doubt, and to find small, unexpected moments of strength along the way. They are about the battles I fought quietly, the lessons that surfaced in the silence, and the gradual realization that sometimes the hardest part of medicine is not treating others, but learning to believe in yourself.

That feeling of inadequacy did not teach me humility — it taught me perspective. For as I kept going, I came to see that success in medicine was not a finish line; it was something else entirely: it's where the journey begins — with self-doubt, sacrifice, and the fight to believe in yourself.

The Backdrop and the Beginning

Boston has always been more than a city to me. It is the backdrop of my childhood, the compass that set my direction, and the place where ambition first found its footing. It is where I learned how the quiet stability of roots can coexist with the restless pull of dreams.

Boston was the rhythm of my coming of age. The smell of Dunkin' Donuts coffee on a chilly morning, the rattle of the commuter rail pulling into North Station, the way the Charles River glittered under late autumn light — all of it carried a pulse that seemed to whisper possibility.

I grew up in Andover, Massachusetts, a small, close-knit community north of Boston. It was the kind of place where you could not walk through the grocery store without seeing someone you knew, where seasons set the rhythm of life. Winter's stillness. Spring's slow thaw. Summer's long evenings. Fall's crisp skies. The crunch of boots on salted sidewalks, the sting of icy wind against skin, and the metallic smell of snow-soaked gloves filled those mornings.

In Andover, you could wake to the sound of birds and be walking the streets of Boston in under an hour. We were close enough to feel Boston's pulse, but far enough to keep our own quiet charm. Teachers knew your parents, and parents knew your friends. The town had two middle schools, but they might as well have been in different countries. We knew the other kids, but not really. They stuck to themselves, and we stuck to ours — two small worlds moving in parallel.

Winters meant trudging down icy sidewalks before sunrise, waiting at the bus stop while snowflakes stung your cheeks and your breath hung in the air like smoke. Those mornings taught me patience, resilience, and the quiet camaraderie of a shared shiver with friends.

I attended public school in Andover through middle school, where I made the kind of friendships that define who you think you are at that age: loyal, formative, and inseparable. The playgrounds were metal swings and blacktop courts, the soccer fields worn at the goal mouths.

High school pulled me further out. I attended Lawrence Academy in Groton, Massachusetts, an hour's drive that felt like a small act of independence. Each morning, winding through back roads before sunrise, I was already learning discipline: balancing classes, sports, and the demands of a place that expected you to give more than you thought you had. Fall meant football games under skies sharp with the smell of leaves and concession-stand popcorn; winter meant early morning or late night hockey practices and long drives with my brother, back and forth to school no matter the weather — snow piling on the roads, windshield wipers working overtime, and the quiet satisfaction of knowing we'd make it there and back.

Still, Boston was never far from my mind. On weekends, I would slip into the city, drawn to its mix of history and momentum. Walking out of North Station or stepping off the Green Line felt like entering another world — horns blaring, street conversations spilling into the air, the city's energy pushing you forward.

Cambridge buzzed with students and ideas, brick paths leading past coffee shops where you could feel smarter just by sitting down. Faneuil Hall's cobblestones echoed with street performers' music, while the harbor carried a salty breeze that promised fresh lobster rolls. South Boston had its grit and pride; Beacon Hill had its gas-lit elegance. Passing Massachusetts General Hospital, I saw the building as the pinnacle of medicine — never knowing how closely my life would one day be tied to that world.

And then there was Northeastern University — the true turning point where I would meet the love of my life, Farah. She was my girlfriend then and my wife now. Whenever Farah and I return to Boston, we walk through campus. For us, it is more than nostalgia; it is a time capsule. Late-night study sessions. Sprinting across Huntington Avenue in the rain. Hockey games at Matthews Arena. Long hours in the library. The low rumble of the Green Line beneath my feet and the damp chill of rain-soaked textbooks pressed against my chest remain etched in memory.

Just a few blocks away was 95 Gainsborough Street, where Farah and her brother lived, where countless conversations stretched into the early morning, and where friendship turned into something more. It's where my initial thought of pursuing medical school came about. I knew Boston before the Big Dig reshaped its streets, before the skyline was nothing more than the Hancock and Prudential towers, or so I thought. I knew it when the Boston Garden was the place to be — before it lost the "Garden" and became something sleeker, shinier, and somehow less intimate. That was my Boston. The one that felt gritty and unpolished in the best way.

Looking back, Boston taught me two things that have shaped each chapter since: Andover gave me roots, but Boston gave me wings — and medicine taught me how to use them.

The leap from the familiar streets of Andover and the bustling energy of the city into the uncertainty of medical training was both thrilling and humbling. I carried with me the discipline of early mornings, the resilience of icy bus stops, and the quiet confidence that came from navigating two worlds — one grounded, one in constant motion. Medicine would test all of it. The leap from familiar streets into the crucible of medical training was more than a change of scenery; it was a test of identity, resilience, and purpose.

The Marrow of Medicine

From my Boston roots, the journey continued into medical training, where self-doubt and resilience became daily truths. The marrow of medicine is not in answers. There have been times in my life when I have had no choice but to pivot.

I can still remember the weight of the beeper on my hip — the dread it would go off again before I had even finished the last page of notes. It wasn't just exhaustion; it was the gnawing fear that maybe I wasn't cut out for this. That fear became my shadow, following me into each patient room until I finally learned to pivot, to adapt, to survive. And you don't need a white coat to know this feeling. Everyone has lived their own crucible — those seasons where exhaustion and self-doubt press in, yet you keep going.

In the middle of the night, the hospital carried an uneasy stillness. Hallways dim, conversations hushed, the air heavy with waiting. The silence never lasted long. A code announcement fractured it, or the phone jolted me with another admission. I came to know the rhythm: sudden bursts of urgency, the rattle of a supply cart, the clipped footsteps of a nurse hurrying past, then again — the hollow quiet that followed.

It was in that quiet, not the noise, that I felt the weight of medicine most. Alone with my thoughts, fatigue sharpened into questions: Had I missed something? Did I order the right test? Could I be trusted with responsibility that felt larger than me? Residency wasn't only about learning medicine; it was about learning to carry doubt, to sit with uncertainty, and still move forward.

At three in the morning, pen in hand, trying to write clearly while my body begged to collapse, I realized residency was not just training — it was a crucible. It shaped not only what I knew, but who I was becoming.

Finding the Way Forward

Waiting for others to decide my path was its own kind of paralysis. In medicine and in life, progress comes not from waiting, but from continuing to move — even when the way forward feels uncertain.

I have come to understand that the first opportunity presented isn't always the best one — and sometimes it's not the right one at all. You can't build your life on someone else's timetable. Their urgency may not match yours. Their priorities may be different. And that's okay — but you can't let that stall you.

Patience is a virtue, but it can also be a trap if it turns into passivity. Yes, we need to wait for the right opportunities to unfold, but waiting shouldn't mean standing still. Keep pushing forward, keep exploring, keep opening doors. There is always more than one path.

One of the hardest things to accept in medicine is that the timeline you want isn't always the one you get. You study for years with a clear vision of how your career will unfold — medical school, residency, fellowship, attending physician — each step neatly aligned with effort and preparation. And then reality interrupts that plan.

You might not match into the specialty you dreamed about. You might match, but not where you hoped to train. You might spend an extra year strengthening an application, repeating boards, or reconsidering a path you once thought was certain. Some physicians enter practice later than expected. Others pivot specialties entirely. The timeline you imagined quietly shifts, sometimes without warning.

In medicine, we are trained to believe that preparation guarantees progression. Yet careers in this field rarely move in straight lines. The match process, board exams, fellowship selection, and even job opportunities introduce variables that no amount of planning can fully control. The hardest lesson is learning that delay does not mean failure. Sometimes it simply means your career is unfolding in a way you did not anticipate — but one that may ultimately shape you into a more thoughtful, resilient physician.

It's human nature to want closure. We want answers so we can move forward. Yet life rarely works in neat, predictable timelines. That uncertainty can be excruciating — especially for people who are used to controlling their schedules and making quick decisions.

The danger is when waiting turns into paralysis. We tell ourselves: I'll make my next move when I hear back. Yet sometimes, that day doesn't come. Or it comes with an answer we didn't expect, and in the meantime, we've lost momentum.

I have learned that the best way to guard against this paralysis is to refuse to stop moving. Even if I'm waiting for one answer, I'm pursuing another opportunity. If a door hasn't opened yet, I'm already knocking on the next one.

Never rely on a single outcome. Always have options on the table. When you do, you give yourself freedom. You remove the power of disappointment because you're not all-in on one uncertain thing. You create space for flexibility — and flexibility is where real confidence grows.

In medicine, we call it having a "backup plan." If the first treatment doesn't work, you already know your second step.

When Timelines Don't Match

The most challenging part of waiting is realizing that what you want and what someone else wants might not line up. Maybe they have other priorities. Maybe their process takes longer than you think it should. Maybe they don't feel the same urgency as you do.

It's not personal; it's reality.

Still if you're used to being on your own schedule, it can feel personal. You can start to wonder if you're being ignored or overlooked. You can start to take it as a reflection of your worth. The truth? It rarely is. Most of the time, their delay says more about their process than about your value. That's why it's so important to stay focused on your own path. You can acknowledge their timeline without letting it control yours.

The best antidote to anxious waiting is focused action. Keep your mind occupied with goals that move you forward — goals you set for yourself, not ones dictated by someone else's timeline. That could mean starting a side project, developing a new skill, networking with people in your field, or working toward personal goals like fitness or family time.

When you have a clear prize in mind, you protect your spirit from the erosion of uncertainty. You remind yourself that your worth isn't determined by one person's decision or one company's offer. Positive action breeds positive thoughts, and positive thoughts protect both your soul and your ambition.

Opportunities will come and go. Some doors will open quickly, others slowly, and some not at all, yet as long as you keep moving, you'll always be ready when the right one appears. Wait for answers when you have to, yet keep building your options. Keep setting new goals. Keep moving forward.

The truth is, the most important decision isn't the one someone else makes about you. It's the one you make about yourself — whether to keep going, to adapt, to pivot, and to believe that your story is still being written.

A Different Kind of Education

Not all growth comes from adapting or pushing forward. Some truths reveal themselves through tears, through loneliness, through the weight of medicine's emotional cost. Painful as they were, moments like those marked the beginning of my deeper education.

This was where medicine stopped being an abstract ambition and became a test of spirit. I learned not only how to cry, but how to rise again. That emotional curriculum became my truest education — and it has never left me.

What textbooks couldn't teach, those nights of unraveling did. They taught me that vulnerability is not weakness, but proof that we are still alive to what matters. They reminded me that the work is not just about knowledge or stamina, but about how much of yourself you are willing to bring into the room. And they forced me to reckon with the truth that healing others will always require finding a way to keep healing yourself.

That was the shift: From memorizing medicine to inhabiting it. From chasing certainty to shouldering its absence. From surviving the grind to learning how to live within it. It was in those fragile, formative moments that I began to glimpse what kind of doctor — and what kind of human being — I might become.

Before I mastered the mechanics of medicine, I was already learning how to carry its weight — not in a hospital residency or an exam room, but in medical school, where the relentless rhythm of long study days and late-night charting, the distance from home, and the relentless uncertainty began shaping me in ways I hadn't anticipated.

Every doctor learns anatomy, physiology, and pathology. Those are the foundations. Yet, no syllabus ever outlined the emotional education that came alongside them.

I didn't go the traditional route. I trained in the Caribbean, far from the safety net of home. While my peers in the States had access to support systems, familiarity, and geographical comfort, I was thousands of miles away from my family, my girlfriend, and my roots. Everything that grounded me was suddenly out of reach.

The sticky salt air clung to skin, ceiling fans chopped through humid silence, and sudden rains hammered tin rooftops during lectures. My own doubts echoed louder than the surf outside.

Medical school is often described as a grind, and that's accurate, but it doesn't quite capture the emotional toll. For me, it was an isolating, disorienting, and emotionally relentless experience.

Getting to class required physical effort. Getting off the island required a logistical miracle. There were no quick weekend trips home, no spontaneous meetups with friends, no chance to decompress with the familiar. I was alone with my ambition. And at times, it felt less like a guiding light and more like a heavy anchor pulling me under.

It was about how I would respond to self-doubt, to fear, to loneliness. I didn't yet realize it, but this was my first introduction to the emotional curriculum of medicine.

And yet, in that isolation, I began to notice something I had never fully recognized before: Medicine wasn't about how many pathways I could memorize or how many practice questions I could complete. Medicine was not going to challenge me intellectually, but emotionally.

There wasn't one dramatic collapse, one single day when everything fell apart. Instead, it was a slow accumulation — a thousand tiny moments that eventually spilled over. The exhaustion of endless study days. The sting of disappointing exam scores. The phone calls home that ended too quickly, with me pretending I was fine. The silence of an empty room at the end of another 14-hour day.

I remember sitting at my desk late one night, notes scattered in front of me, staring at material I had read a dozen times but couldn't seem to absorb. My chest felt heavy, my head pounded, and then, without warning, the tears came — not quiet, controlled tears, but the kind that break through when you've been holding too much for too long.

At first, I kept it together. I told myself this was normal, that everyone went through it. Yet over time, the cracks began to show.

I cried for the distance. I cried for the fear of failure. I cried for the version of myself I thought I was losing — the one who loved medicine, who had once been so certain of his path. At that moment, I wasn't a future physician. I was a young man wondering if he had made a mistake, if he belonged, if he was enough.

That night didn't change everything at once, yet it was the beginning of a shift. For the first time, I acknowledged that I couldn't muscle my way through medical school on discipline alone. I had to learn how to sit with uncertainty, how to find strength in small victories, and how to accept that medicine was going to demand as much from my heart as from my head.

Learning the Hard Lessons

As the years passed, I began to recognize patterns in the way medicine educated me. Some truths came in moments of triumph — passing an exam I thought I might fail, successfully presenting on rounds, or finally feeling like I could contribute something meaningful to a patient's care — yet many of the most important truths came in the quiet, painful spaces.

I learned resilience not in grand victories but in getting back up after disappointing setbacks. I learned humility when I came to see I couldn't possibly know everything, no matter how many hours I studied. I learned vulnerability in the late-night conversations with classmates where we admitted our fears, and for a brief moment, we didn't feel so alone.

Most importantly, I learned to carry the weight of my emotions without letting them crush me. I discovered that fear could be a teacher, that doubt could sharpen rather than paralyze me, and that tears were not a sign of weakness but of engagement — they meant I cared enough to be affected.

By the time I entered residency and, later, independent practice, the emotional terrain of medicine looked different. Gone were the days of crying in solitude about whether I belonged. The challenges became more external, more real, more connected to the lives of others. Now, it's the passing of a long-time patient, the grief etched into a daughter's face when her father slips away. It's the pause before walking into a room to deliver news that will alter the course of a family's life. It's the unexpected moment when a patient says, "I trust you with my life," and you feel the gravity of what that means.

These moments don't test your medical knowledge; they test your humanity. They ask you to be steady when the ground feels unsteady, to be present when words are inadequate, to hold space for emotions that can't be solved with a prescription.

And outside of medicine, the same is true. No manual teaches you how to face loss, heartbreak, or uncertainty. We all improvise through the hardest parts of life.

There is no textbook chapter on how to sit with a grieving family. No multiple-choice question prepares you for telling a mother her child isn't coming back. These are truths only lived experience can teach, and yet, when they arrive, you find yourself reaching back — not to the neat diagrams of medical school, but to the emotional foundation you've been building all along.

The Hidden Curriculum

Looking back, I don't regret the breakdowns or the isolation of those early years. In fact, I see them now as essential. Those nights of doubt, those tears behind closed doors, were not signs of weakness; they were part of my education.

They taught me that resilience is not the absence of struggle but the willingness to face it. They showed me that compassion requires first acknowledging your own vulnerability. They reminded me that presence — being with someone in their hardest moments — is sometimes the most important act of medicine.

Those struggles teach you, in ways large and small, that being a doctor means being both human and healer at the same time.

This is the hidden curriculum no professor ever outlines: That medicine is not only about healing bodies but also about carrying the emotional weight that comes with it. It asks you to diagnose disease, yes, but also to diagnose yourself — to notice when you're weary, when you're overwhelmed, when you need to reset.

And so, when I think back to those first tears in medical school, I no longer see them as failure. I see them as the beginning of my true education.

I remember staring at a stack of anatomy flashcards that refused to make sense, the lines of muscle and nerve blurring together. I remember walking out of an exam convinced I didn't belong, my hands still shaking from scribbling answers I wasn't sure of. I remember a patient encounter where I froze, unable to find the right words, the silence stretching longer than it should have.

And somewhere in those moments, the tears came — not from weakness, but from the weight of realizing how much this work would ask of me.

The science of medicine can be memorized. The protocols can be rehearsed. But the part of medicine with no ICD code — the part measured in presence, vulnerability, and humanity — can only be lived. It is learned moment by moment, tear by tear, patient by patient. Those tears were not weakness. They were initiation. They marked the first time I understood that being a doctor was not about erasing your humanity, but about carrying it into the work.

That has been, and continues to be, the most important lesson of all.

The Weight of What We Miss

We talk a lot about excellence in medicine — about accuracy, precision, perfection. It's baked into our training, our expectations, our daily habits. It's not what we aim for; it's what's assumed of us. From the first day of medical school, there's an unspoken belief: If you work hard enough, if you study enough, if you care enough, you'll get it right.

Still that's not how it works. Not because we're reckless, not because we don't care, but because we're human.

Sometimes what we miss is small. A borderline lab value. A minor complaint tucked into a conversation about bigger issues. A hesitation in someone's voice. Things that don't demand immediate action but quietly ask for it. Other times it's not even a matter of oversight — it's timing. Something hadn't declared itself yet. The symptoms were vague. The story wasn't ready to unfold.

Even when the outcome wasn't devastating, even when the chart is technically "clean," even when no one else would've done anything differently, we ask ourselves the question that never really leaves: Did I do enough?

This is the part of medicine we don't talk about enough: the weight of what we miss.

There's a peculiar type of guilt that comes from knowing that although you did everything right by the book, it wasn't enough. Maybe the patient didn't improve. Maybe their trust in the system cracked. Maybe they never came back to your practice. These aren't the kinds of outcomes you find in outpatient clinical guidelines, but they're the ones that live in the back of your mind.

I've built rituals around this discomfort. At the end of the day, before I leave my office, I scroll through each patient I saw. I read over my notes again. I make sure no labs were missed, no orders forgotten, no subtle concern brushed aside. Some might call it obsessive, yet for me, it's survival. It's the only way I can leave the office and sleep with a somewhat quiet mind.

Was that cough just a lingering cold? Should I have done more for that vague fatigue? Did I brush off that chest pain too quickly? These are the questions that follow us home, echoing long after the clinic doors close.

They don't debilitate me anymore. But they sit at the edge of my consciousness — a constant hum that reminds me I'll never be perfect, that this work, for all its meaning, will never offer total control or complete clarity. And we do our best to put them together into something whole, something true, to become so thorough, so vigilant, so skilled that nothing could slip through.

Now I carry the truth: The goal isn't perfection — it's presence. It's staying engaged, staying humble, staying willing to question and re-question what you thought you knew.

That doesn't mean we stop striving. We owe our patients our best — our sharpest thinking, our most focused attention, our full hearts. Still, we also have to accept the limits of what even our best can do. For even when we do everything right, outcomes don't always align. Sometimes they disappear, and we're left wondering why.

There are patients I'll never forget — not because I made a critical error, but because I couldn't make the difference I so badly wanted to make. I couldn't alter the trajectory. I couldn't break through the noise or uncertainty or complexity of their situation. Sometimes they weren't ready; sometimes I wasn't ready either.

The burden isn't clinical — it's emotional. It's knowing you poured yourself into someone and came up short. It's seeing someone slip through the cracks, despite your efforts to catch them. It's showing up again the next day with that same effort, that same care, knowing it could happen again.

The longer I practice, the more I realize that this is the quiet cost of caring, a kind of cumulative mourning — for the things we couldn't fix, for the stories we couldn't rewrite. And in that word — practicing — there's an uncomfortable truth: It's a craft we'll never perfect.

We're learning in real time, with real people. There's no simulation. No pause button, No redo.

The system doesn't make this easier. We miss things not because we're human, but because the structure around us is flawed. We can't always give each patient the time they deserve. And when we can't, we're the ones who carry that burden home.

I used to think the "good" doctors didn't have doubts, that once you knew enough, you could move through your day with confidence and clarity. Now I understand that the best doctors are the ones who never stop questioning themselves, who accept the messiness of human health and show up with compassion. The best doctors are not defined by answers. They are remembered for their presence — willing to keep searching, even when the answers don't come easily.

And even when we can't solve it entirely, we can bear witness. We can offer care that's thoughtful, intentional, human. Some we'll find too late; some we'll never find at all.

Let's Start at the Beginning

There's a version of medicine you learn in textbooks — and then there's the one you live. Medical education is built on steppingstones. From the MCAT to board exams, each phase is designed to assess your readiness, yet in truth, most of what shapes you as a doctor happens outside the pages of any textbook. It's the hidden curriculum — the unwritten, unspoken truths you pick up along the way — that teaches you how to be a real physician.

The MCAT. My opinion? Antiquated. I understand the need for a standardized metric — a way to sort through thousands of applicants — but I don't believe it captures what truly makes a good doctor. It measures memorization, test-taking strategy, and endurance. What it doesn't measure is empathy, resilience, or the ability to sit with a patient's pain.

I barely remember the test itself — only the hours of tutoring sessions and prep courses I'm not sure made much difference. My score didn't feel like it reflected me, and I doubt I'm alone in that. Still, there had to be a process, and this was it. We play the game because it's the only one offered.

I'm not faulting admissions committees; it's a tough job. But the process often strips away the context of a candidate's journey. I never felt like my full story was fully considered. Still, I got into medical school, and once I did, I discovered medical school to be both brutally challenging and, to my surprise, deeply enjoyable. Because in the end, the admissions process, with all its complexity, boils down to numbers: grades, test scores, and whatever story you can squeeze into a personal statement. It reduces years of resilience, setbacks, and growth into a few lines on a transcript. It can't capture the long nights of doubt, the detours that shape you, or the fire that keeps you pressing forward when no one is watching.

Then comes medical school. Suddenly the numbers don't matter as much. What matters is stamina, curiosity, humility, and the willingness to learn from failure. The abstract ambition of becoming a doctor turns into something tangible: dissecting cadavers, memorizing pathways, fumbling through first patient encounters. It's no longer about proving you belong; it's about learning how to.

It was a constant uphill climb, but we were climbing together. We learned anatomy, pharmacology, physiology — foundational knowledge that built the scaffolding of our understanding. Was any of it real medicine? Not quite. Yet it was necessary. The cadaver lab, the pharmacokinetics, the endless PowerPoints were all part of the process, however removed it felt from the bedside. Those first two years were a blur of lectures, flashcards, and survival. We all struggled.

It wasn't until outpatient clinical rotations that medicine started to feel real. Was it glamorous? Absolutely not. Yet it was transformative. You start to see the human side of medicine: the nuance, the emotion, the unpredictability. You fumble through your presentations. You question whether you belong, and slowly, you build confidence. Those rotations give you a taste of each specialty, a chance to see what fits and what doesn't. For me, internal medicine made sense. It aligned with how I think, how I connect, and how I wanted to grow.

The first time I rounded on patients with a real attending, I remember thinking: This is it. This is what I signed up for. Matching into residency was a milestone I will never forget. It wasn't just the next step in training — it was the doorway into becoming the kind of physician I had worked so hard to be.

I was fortunate to train under leaders who looked past résumés and test scores, past the hierarchy and posturing that so often define medicine. They weren't impressed by where you went to school or how high your Step score was. What they valued was potential, humility, the willingness to learn, and the ability to grow. They saw people, not pedigrees. And for that, I will always be grateful.

The best mentors carried themselves with a quiet authority — the kind that didn't need to raise its voice to be respected. They taught with patience, but also with expectation. They held us accountable, demanded enough to stretch us, but never so harshly as to break us.

From them I learned that medicine is as much about listening as it is about knowing. That a physician's credibility doesn't come from the letters after a name, but from the presence you bring to the bedside.

Residency was grueling — long nights, endless admissions, exhaustion that seeped into your bones. But within that grind lived the most important lessons: that humility opens doors knowledge alone cannot, that presence often matters more than perfection, and that who you are as a doctor is inseparable from who you are as a human being.

Lessons Beyond Medicine

The first code I ever ran came at three in the morning. I walked into the room, a fresh MD just starting residency, and suddenly all eyes were on me. The pressure was unmistakable: A life hung in the balance, and I was expected to lead.

My hands trembled as I called out for chest compressions and epinephrine, my voice higher than I wanted it to be. The monitor flickered — flat line, a spike, then nothing. For a moment, it felt like the whole room was holding its breath. We didn't get him back.

I stepped into the quiet hallway, the echo of the code still buzzing in my ears. Sweat clung to my scrubs. My pulse refused to slow. I had memorized algorithms, rehearsed scenarios, but nothing prepared me for the gravity of a life ending under my watch.

That night taught me what no textbook could: Medicine is not just steps on a flowchart; it's finding your voice in chaos. It's staying present when the outcome slips beyond your control. It was my first glimpse of the unbridgeable space between knowledge and humanity — and the realization that carrying that space would be part of the work forever.

Those three years were transformative. I learned more than medicine; I learned humility in the face of uncertainty, patience in the process of becoming, and resilience when exhaustion blurred the days into nights. Residency taught me how to manage illness, yes, but more importantly, it taught me how to carry the responsibility of being present for another human being. What I absorbed in those years shaped not only the doctor I would become, but the person.

I learned how to deliver bad news with grace. I learned what it meant to stay up all night worrying about a patient, even when no one was watching. I learned that medicine is as much about knowing when to speak as it is about knowing when to listen.

We had a team that supported one another. We weren't arrogant; we were earnest. We wanted to learn, to help. And, above all, we wanted to become the kind of doctors our patients deserved. It wasn't about managing complex cases or presenting on rounds. It was about how you carry yourself during a code.

That's the thing most people don't realize: You become a doctor long before the title becomes official. You graduate. You're an attending. And then, like that, it's over. There's no one signing off your orders anymore. There's no one double-checking your plans. You're the final word.

No one teaches you how to manage a full outpatient clinic schedule, navigate billing systems, or run a multidisciplinary team. No one teaches you how to support your staff or respond to angry phone calls from patients or families. You're expected to know how to do all of it because you carry the title now, yet so much of it is learned through trial by fire.

You realize quickly that medicine isn't just about diagnostics or disease management. It's about communication. It's about cultural sensitivity. It's about adapting — sometimes by the hour. I had to learn how to care for patients from every background, how to pivot when plans unraveled, and how to sit with the discomfort of not having clear answers.

None of that is in *Harrison's* or any other textbook. That's not theory; it's real life.

Yes, I had excellent training, yet the real practice of medicine happens after the training wheels come off. And it's in that space — the vulnerable, high-stakes, emotionally charged space — that you figure out who you are as a doctor.

I learn something new every day. That's another truth of the hidden curriculum: You're never done, you're never perfect, and that's okay. What matters is that you show up. That you care. That you listen. That you try.

So much of what makes a great doctor has nothing to do with what you memorize; it's about how you make someone feel. It's about trust, about presence, about humility. The textbooks will always be there. They'll evolve with time. Yet the hidden curriculum — the real education — that's something you only earn by living it. And I wouldn't trade that for anything.

Intimidation to Invitation

One of the most important — and least discussed — truths in medicine is this: Feeling inadequate in medicine isn't rare; it's everywhere — quiet, lingering, relentless.

Two patients on the schedule — one before lunch and one after — and still my palms sweated as if I were about to step onto a stage before an auditorium full of people. I reread each chart three times, terrified of missing something small that might matter. Those early days weren't defined by efficiency or confidence; they were defined by survival.

Yet slowly, as more faces began to appear, something shifted. Each day brought new patients — strangers who walked in with their stories, their fears, and their trust. I no longer saw just charts and chief complaints; I saw lives unfolding in front of me. What once felt like intimidation began to feel like invitation.

Fear gave way to familiarity. Anxiety gave way to trust. And with each new patient, I realized that medicine was never about perfection. It was about presence — the simple, steady act of showing up for whoever sat across from me.

The first day I stepped into the outpatient clinic as an attending, I was struck by the smell: the unmistakable mix of antiseptic wipes, alcohol swabs, printer ink, and brewed coffee that had been sitting too long. My name was on every chart. I had my own office, a computer, even an office chair — ordinary things I once thought were too big for me.

And still, it felt almost fraudulent, as if I were slipping into a costume I hadn't earned, sitting in a seat meant for someone else. The white coat was mine, the title was mine, but the certainty? That still belonged to someone I was trying to become.

I had started my outpatient practice right out of residency, joining a large multispecialty group, surrounded by physicians who had trained at top-tier institutions and carried résumés that spoke for themselves. Many had been practicing for decades, their reputations well established, their patient panels already full.

And then there was me: newly minted, still learning to trust my own judgment, with a panel that began at zero. The gulf between us felt wide. Yet it was in that space — between inexperience and expectation — that I began to discover the kind of doctor I wanted to become. They were confident, efficient, experienced. I was waiting on my board scores, unsure if I was even certified yet. And yet there I was, seeing patients. Trying to find my footing. Surrounded by colleagues who felt light years ahead of me.

They had full panels; I had two or three patients a day. They flew through the EMR; I could barely open a note. They had systems; I had questions — endless questions. Was I writing my notes the right way? Had I overlooked something important? What if a patient didn't like me — or worse, what if they complained about me? Every interaction felt like a test, and I was never sure if I was passing.

I stayed late after clinic, rewriting notes that probably didn't need rewriting, second-guessing every phrase, every order, every plan. I reread lab results long after the patient had gone home, searching for something I might have missed. Even a normal visit could leave me replaying conversations on the drive home, dissecting every word for signs of failure.

The pressure wasn't just about being right; it was about being trusted. A single chart carried someone's story, someone's fear, someone's future. And while my colleagues down the hall seemed to move effortlessly through their schedules, I felt like I was learning to walk again, every step uncertain and unsteady.

Yet, with each patient who returned, each follow-up that confirmed I hadn't missed the mark, the ground grew a little steadier beneath me. What began in fear slowly started to look like belonging.

And what I have come to understand since is this: Inadequacy isn't a new physician's burden; it lingers, even in the most seasoned among us. All it takes is a bad outcome, a tough patient, a complaint. Suddenly, the confidence you worked so hard to build is shaken.

In medicine, starting something new — whether it's your first job or your fifth — isn't just a transition; it's a rebuild. You're not simply adding your name to a clinic roster or stepping into a new system. You're rebuilding from the ground up: a patient panel, a foundation of trust, and a rhythm that's sustainable — not only for your patients, but for yourself.

Everything to Everyone

When I left residency, I had logged thousands of hours managing hospitalized patients — rounding, running codes, responding to emergencies. But outpatient medicine? That was an entirely different world.

I had to learn how to use the EMR without drowning in it. How to fit structure into a 15-minute visit without making patients feel rushed. How to guide prevention and lifestyle change in ways that felt realistic, not rehearsed. How to communicate uncertainty without losing trust. And above all, how to earn that trust in the first place.

It doesn't happen overnight. It takes time to earn patients' trust — and even longer to trust yourself. It can take years before patients open up, before they believe in you, before they refer their friends and family. And in that in-between — when your panel is light and your confidence is low — inadequacy creeps in.

We're human. We want to be respected, to do right by our patients, to feel like we're doing a good job. And when we don't, we internalize it — not as a mistake, but as a flaw. Many of us carry a dangerous belief: That we should be excellent at everything, all the time — not only great clinicians, but great partners, great parents, great friends, great leaders. And when we fall short — even just a little — we don't brush it off. We feel it deeply.

It isn't just doubt; it's a pit in your stomach, a voice that whispers: You should know this. You should be better by now.

In medicine, mistakes carry weight. A missed diagnosis isn't a slip — it can be life-changing. A delayed test isn't a clerical error — it can be costly. That pressure never disappears. And when it mixes with the emotional weight we carry for our patients, it can feel overwhelming.

Still, here's what I wish more of us knew sooner: That feeling is normal. In fact, the physicians who care the most often carry the heaviest sense of inadequacy because they care deeply. They worry about outcomes. They want to excel because they know what's at stake.

But no one — not even the most seasoned among us — can be excellent at every moment. Trying to be everything for everyone leads only to burnout and self-doubt. You don't have to be everything at all at once. You are allowed to build slowly. Balance will come with time. Confidence doesn't arrive in a single moment; it grows quietly through repetition, humility, and persistence. And even then, just when you start to feel steady, something new will challenge you. That's not failure; that's proof you're still in the game, still learning, still caring, still showing up.

Yes, the boat will rock. Some days you'll feel like you're sinking. But most days, you'll find your balance. And that is what makes a great physician: not perfection, but persistence; not certainty, but commitment.

You are not alone. You are not inadequate. You are not failing. You are worthy of the degree you earned, the role you hold, and the life you're building. Find your lane. Do your best. Be kind to yourself. And trust that confidence will come — not all at once, but quietly, over time, through grace and the work you continue to do.

Brick by Brick

When I began this journey, I thought success was a finish line — that if I worked hard enough, studied long enough, and sacrificed deeply enough, I'd finally cross it. I pushed through sleepless nights in college. Carried relentless pressure in medical school. Survived the blur of residency, where days and nights dissolved into each other. I lived with my eyes fixed on the horizon — on the next exam, the next rotation, the next milestone.

And in doing so, I missed something important: I was so focused on who I was becoming that I forgot to value who I already was.

If I could speak to that version of myself, I'd tell him this: Know your worth. Own your value. Stand tall in your growth. Set expectations by your experience — not someone else's standards. Set expectations by your progress — not someone else's pace.

Success isn't luck. It isn't given. It's built brick by brick — through hard work, smart choices, deep relationships, and a kind of grit that refuses to quit. And the truth is, you don't learn that from winning; you learn it from failing, from adapting, from rising again.

At some point, I stopped chasing the version of success I thought I was supposed to want and started chasing the life I was meant to live. I stopped apologizing for my ambition. I trusted my instincts because they had carried me further than fear ever could. And that's when everything began to change.

Over time, I came to see that becoming a doctor is a path admired by many but walked by few. It demands more than intelligence; it demands empathy, resilience, humility. And if you're not careful, it can take so much of you that you forget to live the life you're building it for.

Looking back now, I understand that life is short. Cherish the people who stand beside you, not behind you. It's not about how many are in your corner, but about who shows up when it matters. Earn respect, but let only those who've earned yours into your heart.

Don't let one bad moment — or one unkind person — shake your vision. And remember: The finish line always moves. That's the point. Success isn't a destination; it's a journey.

It's hard. Accept that. Yet define what fulfillment means to you — not to your mentors, your parents, or society. And if your path leads you to medicine, be the kind of doctor who sees the person before the diagnosis, who listens deeply, who shows up fully, who remembers what it felt like to sit on the other side of the stethoscope.

That is the kind of physician who earns lifelong respect — and the kind of person who leaves behind a legacy that matters. My path wasn't the traditional one, but it was mine. I took a different route to pursue my dream, and that route carried me far from the familiar — to an island hundreds of miles from home, where the heat pressed down, the trade winds carried salt through the air, and my classmates and I quickly learned that this would not be the glossy version of medical school we had imagined. It was humbling, disorienting, and exactly where my journey had to begin.

There were moments I truly wondered if I'd make it. I was afraid I'd fail — that this dream might slip through my fingers. How could I study medicine on a tiny island and be taken seriously as a doctor in the United States?

I turned to forums like ValueMD for comfort, desperate to read the words of someone who had walked this road before me. I scoured pages on KevinMD and Student Doctor Network, searching for reassurance that this path could lead somewhere — that I wasn't alone, that others had started from the same uncertain place and still found their way. For at the time, I had little else to hold on to.

The Path in Detail

Getting into a U.S. medical school is brutally competitive. Each year, thousands of bright, passionate students are turned away — not because they're unqualified, but because there aren't enough spots. Meanwhile, our country faces a worsening physician shortage. We need more doctors, not fewer. That's where Caribbean medical schools come in and, unfortunately, that's also where the stigma begins.

There's a persistent myth in medicine: If you went to school outside the United States — especially in the Caribbean — you must be less capable, less prepared, somehow less worthy.

That myth is wrong. I'm living proof — and so are countless others. We took the same board exams, faced the same standards, and carried the same responsibilities. The path looked different, but the destination — and the commitment — were the same. We completed the same demanding rotations and earned the same licenses to practice medicine.

If you trust the U.S. medical licensing system, then you already trust us because we met the same standards. The difference is that the road from a Caribbean medical school back into the U.S. system isn't a straight path. It's a mountain climb. The steps are steeper, the barriers higher, and the margin for error smaller. But for those who make it, the climb builds something you can't measure on paper: resilience, persistence, and grit.

I've worked shoulder to shoulder with physicians trained all over the world — India, Nigeria, South America, the Caribbean, Europe. And when you're making real-time decisions with real consequences, no one asks where your degree is from. In the chaos of a code, when seconds matter, no one pauses to ask where you trained. In the quiet of an exam room, when a patient is searching your eyes for reassurance, no one cares about the crest on your diploma.

What matters is your knowledge, your instincts, your judgment, your heart. What matters is your ability to stay steady when the room tilts, your willingness to sit with someone's fear without rushing them out the door. That is what patients remember. That is what colleagues respect. That is what saves lives.

I wasn't a tourist in paradise. I was a determined student building a future. Despite the heat, hurricanes, and hardship, I wouldn't trade a minute of it. That was where I became a doctor — where I gained cultural perspective, lifelong friendships, and a resilience I carry with me every day.

Medicine isn't defined by the name stitched on a diploma. It is defined by how you show up when someone's life is on the line. More than a quarter of practicing physicians in the United States are international medical graduates, many trained in the Caribbean. We are not exceptions to the profession. We are part of its foundation.

What most people never see are the details of that path.

I remember sitting in lecture halls where the hum of generators was as familiar as the professor's voice. Storm warnings were not hypothetical conversations — they were part of daily planning. There were days when power outages interrupted lectures mid-sentence, forcing classrooms into sudden stillness before the backup systems flickered on. Studying became an exercise in adaptability. You learned to charge devices whenever electricity was available, to print notes when you could, to prepare for the unexpected because the unexpected was routine.

Outside the classroom, the environment taught its own lessons. Living on an island meant learning to navigate cultural differences, economic disparities, and a healthcare system that looked very different from the one many of us hoped to eventually practice within. That exposure broadened my understanding of medicine long before I fully appreciated its significance. Illness looked different depending on where you lived, what resources you had, and how accessible care truly was. Disease was not only biological; it was social, economic, and cultural.

Clinical training reinforced those lessons. Resources were not always abundant. Advanced imaging or subspecialty consultation was not guaranteed. Physical examination skills were not optional — they were essential. You learned to listen longer, observe more carefully, and trust clinical reasoning in ways that shaped how you approached patient care long after formal training ended. The limitations were not obstacles. They were teachers.

Those experiences didn't weaken my education. They deepened it. They taught me that medicine is not practiced in controlled environments or ideal circumstances. It is practiced in imperfect settings where uncertainty is constant and adaptability is survival. They also taught me humility — the recognition that intelligence alone does not make a physician effective. Perspective, patience, and resilience matter just as much.

That training continues to influence how I practice medicine today. When diagnostic pathways become complicated or resources are delayed, I am less likely to feel paralyzed by those barriers. Instead, I return to the clinical fundamentals that training reinforced — careful listening, thoughtful examination, and a willingness to sit with uncertainty while continuing to move forward.

It also reshaped how I relate to patients navigating unfamiliar or intimidating healthcare environments. I understand what it feels like to work toward a future inside a system that may not fully understand your path or background. That awareness quietly influences how I listen, how I explain, and how I advocate for the people I care for.

That path demanded persistence. It demanded belief when certainty was scarce. I did not arrive in medicine despite where I started. I arrived because I refused to stop moving forward. The training shaped not only the physician I became, but the person I carried into every exam room.

In Retrospect

Looking back, I sometimes feel like I rushed past parts of childhood searching for the next milestone. I focused on proving myself, chasing direction, and trying to define success before I fully understood what success meant to me.

I didn't go out much. I had a small circle of close friends, but I was never part of the popular crowd. At the time, I told myself that didn't matter, and in many ways it didn't. But there were moments when I wondered if I was moving so quickly toward the future that I never fully stopped to understand what I was chasing.

It is difficult to appreciate what you have when you are young. It is even harder to understand what you truly want. We are often taught to pursue external markers of success — financial stability, professional recognition, the symbols that society associates with achievement. Those goals are not inherently wrong, but they are incomplete. Some people ultimately discover that what they crave is simplicity, peace, or purpose. Understanding which of those paths belongs to you is one of life's most difficult and most important challenges.

I don't think I ever had strong self-esteem growing up. It wasn't absent, but it wasn't secure either. Self-worth during those years is fragile. It is shaped not only by family, but by peers, mentors, teachers, coaches, and the people we quietly hope will recognize our potential. Sometimes we look for validation from people who never realize we are searching for it.

It is difficult to feel important. It is difficult to feel seen.

What I carry with me now is a perspective that took years to develop.

Be present. Find happiness in the moment, not just the destination. Discover what energizes you and follow it with courage, even when it feels uncertain or unconventional. Pursue what brings you joy, not simply what earns admiration. The world will always have opinions about success, but only you can define what gives your life meaning.

My younger self stumbled often. I doubted whether I belonged. I questioned my path and faced rejection more than once. But I kept going. I moved forward through setbacks, long nights, exhaustion, and uncertainty. That persistence carried me here — to a place where presence matters more than perfection and fulfillment is measured by the people I serve and the life I have built.

The path was never straight. The plans were never perfect. There was no master strategy guiding it forward. Over time, I learned that overanalyzing rarely produces clarity and overthinking rarely creates peace. Sometimes the most important skill is learning to play the hand you are dealt and trusting that, with time and perspective, that hand may reveal possibilities you never expected.

For years, I lived focused on the future. I planned constantly. I projected forward. I prepared for milestones that always seemed just ahead. In doing so, I sometimes overlooked what was directly in front of me — the present moment quietly passing by.

I am reminded of that lesson every day in my clinic. Patients frequently tell me to enjoy youth, health, and time while they remain available. Many describe their so-called golden years as complicated by illness, responsibility, loss, or physical decline. Their stories serve as daily reminders that life rarely unfolds exactly as we imagine it will.

Those conversations reinforce what I try to practice now: appreciate today. Pursue joy now. Value your health, your time, and your relationships while they are present. The future will arrive whether we are ready or not. This moment only happens once.

Confidence and a True Calling

I remember being in college, sitting with that heavy question: What do I want to do with my life?

I chose medicine. Maybe because I admired doctors. Maybe because I wanted to follow in my father's footsteps. Maybe because my brother went to med school. Maybe because my parents hoped I would. Yet deep down, I knew it had to be my decision.

Many new students and residents think the hardest part is the knowledge, yet what is the biggest challenge? Confidence. When you step into the hospital residency, people start relying on you to make decisions. You'll have attendings and senior residents to guide you, sure, yet to your patients, you are the doctor. That shift is real. That responsibility is heavy, and it brings out the self-doubts: I feared I'd make a mistake, my patients wouldn't like me, I wouldn't do well in my program, I wouldn't match.

We use fear as a defense mechanism. We overthink to protect ourselves from failure, yet most of the time, those fears don't play out; they drain us. Confidence isn't arrogance. Believing in yourself doesn't make you cocky, yet I think too many trainees are afraid to look "too confident," so they tone themselves down and lose the trust in themselves they need to care for others. At the same time, overconfidence without humility is dangerous. So what's the balance?

Believe in yourself — but stay teachable. You don't need to be perfect; you need to show up. Be curious, ask questions, admit when you don't know, and trust that you'll figure it out.

At one point, I thought seriously about becoming a personal trainer. The vision was easy to imagine: I'd move to Hollywood, train celebrities, carve out a good living, and enjoy the perks. It promised freedom, travel, recognition, maybe even glamour. A life built around fitness and performance had its allure — after all, I loved exercise, discipline, and helping others improve themselves.

But when the lights dimmed and the daydreams faded, harder questions always followed. Could I build a future on that? Could I support a family on it? Could I find fulfillment beyond the paycheck and the status?

And the hardest question of all: Would I feel proud of the path when I looked back decades later?

The answer, deep down, was "no." Because what I really wanted wasn't just a job that looked good on the outside — I wanted a vocation that felt meaningful on the inside, a life built not just on aesthetics, but on impact.

Training celebrities might have given me proximity to fame, but it wouldn't give me the sense of calling I was searching for. I didn't want to spend my life counting reps. I wanted to spend it counting moments that mattered — moments in which someone's life changed because I showed up.

That was the difference: Lifestyle versus purpose; perks versus presence; status versus service. And in the end, that's why medicine won. Not because it was easier; not because it was guaranteed. But because it gave me the chance to wake up every morning knowing the work itself carried meaning.

In medical school, I honestly didn't think I'd make it. Every day was a struggle. The tests weren't just exams — they were battles against exhaustion, self-doubt, and the weight of expectation. The competition was everywhere, sometimes spoken, more often unspoken. Everyone seemed smarter, faster, more prepared.

I lived on caffeine and panic. My world shrank to flashcards, highlighters, and the constant hum of fear. I didn't have a life — I had deadlines. Friendships faded. Holidays blurred into study sessions. Birthdays became just another day to memorize pathways and pharmacology.

And beneath it all was fear. Fear that I wouldn't pass. Fear that I would bomb Step 1. Fear that I would never match into residency. The thought looped endlessly: What if all of this — every late night, every sacrifice — was for nothing?

The truth was brutal: A medical degree without board certification isn't a ticket to healing; it's just paper. And the idea of walking away after years of sacrifice with nothing but a framed reminder of failure was unbearable.

That fear lived in my chest like a second heartbeat. It pushed me to study harder, but it also hollowed me out. And for a long time, I wasn't sure which would win. These thoughts consumed me. I carried them like a second backpack — one filled not with books, but with fear, doubt, and self-imposed pressure.

And then came residency, where the fear didn't vanish; it changed shape. Now the stakes were real, boards mattered. Outcomes mattered. Lives depended on my decisions. I doubted myself. Yet slowly, things started to shift — not in big, dramatic ways, but in quiet, steady moments: A friend texting me late at night for medical advice — not because I had the degree, but because they trusted me. A conversation where I didn't have to prove myself because I belonged. Those were the moments I started to feel it: I am a real doctor. Not because I had all the answers, not because I never made mistakes, but because I cared.

I am asked questions all the time by patients, friends, colleagues. And I'm grateful for that — not because it means I carry the truth about everything, but because it means they trust me. They believe in me. And finally, I believe in myself too.

Medicine is evolving fast. Technology, bureaucracy, and burnout are rising. Yet at its core, medicine is about people. It's about connection. It's about showing up with your full, flawed, learning, human self — and being present.

We need more doctors who know how to pause, to listen, to care.

It's okay to question. It's okay to struggle. It's okay to not have it all figured out. You don't need to be the smartest in the room. You don't need to have every answer memorized. What you *do* need is something deeper: to be real.

Be someone who listens. Be someone who leads. Let your voice be your power. Let your purpose be your compass. Let your growth become your story. Because medicine has never been about being perfect. It has always been about becoming whole — and showing up, again and again, for someone who needs you.

That's what real doctors do.

Negative to Positive

I struggle with the persistent negativity around internal medicine. Yes, it's hard. We deal with uncertainty, emotion, and time pressure, yet internal medicine is meaningful, foundational. It's where trust is built. In primary care, you don't just meet patients — you grow up with them, grow old with them. You become part of their story, and they become part of yours. Over the years, the bond shifts from a chart number to a name, from an encounter to a relationship, from a patient to a person you truly know.

One of my first patients was a middle-aged man with uncontrolled diabetes. In those early days, I stumbled through medication adjustments, learning as much from his persistence as he did from my prescriptions. Over the years, I saw him through infections, setbacks, and small victories.

Years later, I walked into the room to find him sitting with his daughter — now a young woman — who wanted me to become her doctor, too. In that moment, I realized continuity isn't just about lab results or medication refills. It's about being present long enough for trust to pass from one generation to the next.

This happens far more often than people realize. A parent entrusts me with their health, and before long, I'm caring for their children — and sometimes their grandchildren, siblings, or extended family. The circle of care widens, not because of contracts or assignments, but because trust extends outward.

Internal medicine is this: showing up long enough to see someone's life arc, to carry their story forward, and to become not just their doctor but part of their family's fabric. That is the privilege and the responsibility that keeps me here.

Patients come to us with everything from vague symptoms to life-altering diagnoses. We walk with them through highs and lows. We become their guides, their advocates, their constant.

You never know what will walk through the door — or what might walk back out. That unpredictability keeps the work sharp, fulfilling, real.

Do I feel pressure? Absolutely. Yet I also feel immense gratitude. The short time I get with patients can make a lifelong impact. That matters.

The system has cracks. Corporate medicine is flawed, yet my team? They're like family. My patients? They trust me. And that trust? It's sacred.

If you're wondering what makes internal medicine worth staying for, this is it:

I walk into clinic never knowing what the day will bring. A routine check-up can become a crisis. A walk-in can turn into a life saved. My hours are filled with chronic conditions, sudden emergencies, shifting priorities, and the endless navigation of personalities and expectations. Yet every day, I get to be more than a doctor. I am a companion, a guide, a steady presence in someone's most vulnerable moments.

To be trusted with that role — to be the person someone turns to when they are scared, when they are hurting, when they need clarity or hope — is a privilege I never take for granted.

I walk with patients through happiness and heartbreak, through disappointments and recoveries, through casual concerns and life-changing diagnoses. I sit with them in tears, in silence, and sometimes in laughter that surprises us both.

Because at the end of the day, patients aren't only reaching out for diagnoses; they're reaching out for reassurance, for perspective, for help carrying the weight of uncertainty. I have become, in some small way, a constant in their chaotic world, and I am profoundly honored by that trust.

What makes it even more meaningful? They've watched me grow, too. When I came out of residency, I wasn't fully prepared for the outpatient world. No one teaches you how to build a practice — how to manage complexity, talk about money, or balance medicine with life. I had to figure it out — sometimes the hard way.

I've faced burnout, difficult encounters, and the tension of juggling work and family. Yet I've also had support from colleagues who believed in me and gave me room to grow. Yes, a few doubted me, but many more lifted me up. Even in a large group, my team and patients feel like family.

I'm grateful. Grateful for the trust, for the relationships, for the chance to do this work every day. I wouldn't change it.

So to the next generation wondering if internal medicine is worth it — if it's fulfilling, if it's sustainable — I say this:

If you're willing to look past the noise — past the metrics and the stress — you'll find something powerful. If you ever need guidance or someone to listen, reach out. We're here. And we'd love to help.

Internal medicine isn't perfect — no specialty is, yet if you focus on the relationships, the meaning, the privilege of caring for others — you'll see what we see. You'll understand why we stay, why we show up, why we believe. And maybe one day, you'll believe in it too.

Medicine doesn't live in textbooks. It lives in the room — where uncertainty, connection, and vulnerability shape every moment. And maybe, just maybe, that's where the real healing begins.

Still sometimes, what defines our work isn't the science; it's the emotional toll, the doubt, and the courage to keep going.

Making Choices

Medical students look at salary charts and prestige rankings and often chase the highest-paying specialties: dermatology, orthopedic surgery, plastic surgery. And while those fields are competitive and impressive in their own right, I wonder how many choose them out of genuine passion — and how many do so for the perceived reward alone.

Primary care has long been viewed by many as a secondary field — less prestigious, less lucrative, less desirable. It's often associated with lower reimbursement, heavy administrative burden, and a lack of control.

This mindset starts in medical school, where we are conditioned to view certain specialties as "elite" and others as fallback options. Primary care is rarely painted as aspirational, yet I think that's misguided.

Primary care is the gateway to medicine. It is the front line, the foundation. It may not always be glamorous, but it is indispensable. It's where most patients begin their journey — and where many relationships in medicine are built.

Yes. Some of the criticisms are true. Reimbursement can be frustrating. Documentation is endless, and patients can be unpredictable — incredibly sweet and occasionally challenging. Yet that's not unique to internal medicine. That's medicine.

What's often overlooked is the versatility of internal medicine. From this one residency, you can launch into nearly any subspecialty. You can pursue outpatient primary care or work exclusively as a hospitalist. You can shift between academic medicine, private practice, public health, and administration. Internal medicine gives you options.

I have no regrets. I love what I do. I love building long-term relationships with my patients. I don't manage one problem; I manage the whole person. I carry the truth of their lives: their stories, their families, their careers, and their struggles. I get to care for the entire human being, not one organ system.

The landscape of medicine is changing. Private equity is creeping in. Hospitals are buying up independent practices. The old model of private practice is fading fast, yet instead of complaining, I adapt. I speak up when needed. I stay quiet when it serves the moment. Most importantly, I stay involved.

I do believe that physicians need a stronger voice in administration. Too often, non-outpatient clinical decision-makers dictate the direction of healthcare without truly understanding the patient experience. Medicine may be a business, but it's a business centered around people, and those of us who care for patients every day need to be at the table when decisions are made.

No matter how far artificial intelligence advances, no matter how many innovations try to replace us, patients want to connect with real people. They want hands-on care, honest conversations, and relationships with someone who listens. A machine may analyze symptoms, but it cannot understand a patient's fear, hesitation, or hope. Only a human can do that.

That's why I believe the future of internal medicine is bright. Internists — whether hospital residency-based or outpatient — remain the backbone of care. We are the ones whom patients turn to first and return to again and again. Our relevance will not fade.

Still, we must push for change. The administrative burden placed on physicians has become overwhelming. Prior authorizations, electronic portals, EMRs, and endless regulations add layers of inefficiency that don't serve the patient or the physician. Some of it may be necessary. Most of it is not.

This is why we need more doctors in leadership. Medicine should be guided by those who understand its soul. Patient care cannot be optimized when physicians are sidelined from the decision-making process. At its core, internal medicine is about connection, complexity, and continuity. It is often undervalued, but never unimportant. And for those of us who love it, there is no better calling.

For too long, primary care has been treated as medicine's "backup plan" — less prestigious, less respected, less desired. It is often seen through a narrow lens: lower pay, higher burden, endless paperwork, unpredictable patients, and little control.

But here's the truth: primary care is not a fallback. It is the foundation. It is the gateway into medicine — the first touchpoint, the steady anchor, the lasting relationship. We don't just manage disease; we manage lives.

We know our patients not only through their medical histories, but through the seasons of their journeys. We know their families, their careers, their fears, their resilience. We treat the person, not the problem.

And that is the privilege of internal medicine.

It asks us to hold the complexity of science alongside the complexity of being human — to walk with people not just through illness, but through life itself.

And we are needed — now more than ever.

Yes, it's hard. Yes, the paperwork is brutal. Yes, the system is deeply flawed. Yet that's not unique to internal medicine. That's the reality of modern healthcare.

What people often miss is the power and versatility of internal medicine. From a single residency, we can go in dozens of different directions. Outpatient care. Inpatient medicine. Subspecialty fellowships. Academic roles. Administrative leadership, Public health. Consulting. Policy. Startups. You name it. Internal medicine opens doors — and I've never once regretted walking through mine.

I love my work. I love the continuity. The relationships. The trust. The ability to guide patients not through illness, but through life. I get to be their adviser, advocate, and partner. That's not a job. That's a privilege.

The future of internal medicine isn't about surviving — it's about evolving. We cannot keep asking physicians to do more with less. Prior authorizations. Pointless portals. Click after click in the EMR. Government regulations that do nothing to improve outcomes. The burdens are crushing, and the people paying the price are the ones who care most: patients and doctors.

True Leadership in Medicine

Medicine has become a business, but it must remain a human one. And that will only happen if more physicians lead. We need doctors — not administrators — at the decision-making table. We need the people who know patient care best shaping the systems that are supposed to support it.

There's no master handbook that tells me precisely what to do for a person who walks into my exam room. Medicine, at its core, is not a series of fixed answers — it's a process of exploration, trust, and adaptation.

We are trained early in medical school to take control, to carry the burden of decision-making. We are taught to lead, to be decisive, to make sound recommendations grounded in evidence and best practice. And that responsibility matters. Patients trust us to know the science and to translate it into action.

But there is a fine line between guiding and dictating. When we slip into the trap of making decisions unilaterally — believing we always know best — we risk something essential: the patient's agency.

Medicine is not a monologue; it is a dialogue. The patient's values, fears, and lived experiences are not footnotes to the clinical plan — they are central to it. When we forget that, we may succeed in treating disease while failing to honor the person living with it.

True leadership in medicine means more than carrying the burden of knowledge; it means sharing the weight of choice, recognizing that healing is not something we deliver to patients, but something we build with them.

And, in some cases, it means distrust. The patient may leave the appointment with a prescription or a test order in hand but feel hesitant, overwhelmed, or unclear about why we chose that course of action. Over time, that uncertainty can grow into anxiety, disengagement, nonadherence, the sense that healthcare is something being done to them, not with them.

Too often, patients are expected to sit back and receive care passively, rather than actively participating in it. This dynamic can lead to misalignment, confusion. That's when medicine stops feeling personal.

Still, when we take the time to sit beside the patient, rather than stand in front of them — when we listen, explore, and collaborate — the entire relationship transforms. Decisions become more meaningful. Plans become more realistic; care becomes more effective.

This doesn't mean we surrender our medical judgment. Quite the opposite. It means we use our knowledge to elevate the conversation, not control it. We bring options to the table: "Here's what I think might help you. Let's talk about what works best for you, given your life, your values, your concerns." We explain risks, benefits, side effects, costs, and we listen to the answers that come back. These conversations, these relationships, are the difference between theoretical medicine and lived medicine.

For example, when choosing a medication, I don't look only at what the guidelines recommend. I consider the patient's prior experiences, allergies, lifestyle, access, and preferences. Is it expensive and not covered well by insurance? Does it come in a form that's easy to swallow or administer? Has the patient had a bad past experience with something similar? These questions matter.

Some patients are decisive. They want to weigh every option, ask every question, and be fully involved in the process. Others feel overwhelmed, uncertain, and quietly hand the responsibility back with words like: "Well, you're the doctor. Just tell me what to do."

In those moments, I remind myself of the balance I owe them. Authority, yes — but never at the cost of partnership. So I answer with care and clarity: "Yes, I'm your doctor, but I'm not here to dictate your health. I'm here to work with you. We'll make this decision together, in a way that works best for you."

Because the truth is, medicine isn't about me making the "right" choice alone. It's about helping patients find the choice that is right for them and walking that path beside them. That partnership builds trust — and trust changes everything.

It means the patient is more likely to understand why we're doing something and, as a result, they are more likely to follow through. They're more comfortable asking questions next time. It opens the door to future conversations, future honesty, future care.

It doesn't take much: a moment of explanation, a pause to invite questions, a recognition that this is their life we're navigating, not our protocol.

There are, of course, times when there is only one reasonable course of action, when delay or indecision could be harmful, but even then, how we communicate matters. Patients are more likely to act on our advice when they feel seen and heard, not instructed.

Shared decision-making doesn't slow us down; it focuses us. It makes our decisions smarter, more personalized, more durable. It reduces unnecessary interventions. It increases satisfaction on both sides. It builds long-term rapport, which is invaluable in primary care and chronic disease management. It turns 15-minute visits into something that feels meaningful, rather than mechanical.

Sometimes I order a test and explain why I think it's important. Other times, I ask, "Would you like to do this now, or wait until the next visit?" There's value in giving space. Autonomy is powerful. Patients appreciate knowing that they have a say, and that I respect their ability to make decisions about their own bodies.

There are certainly patients who prefer the traditional model; they want clear direction and little ambiguity. That's okay, too. Shared decision-making doesn't mean forcing everyone into a philosophical debate. It means being able to read the room, adapt to the individual, and communicate in a way that matches their needs. Some want a map. Others want a compass.

Ultimately, this is what medicine is about: the merging of outpatient clinical insight with human connection. Working as a team. Recognizing that good care isn't about what I think is best — it's about what we decide is best, together.

When we share decisions, we share responsibility. And in doing so, we strengthen the bond that keeps healthcare humane.

The Power of the Selfie

I have a patient who insists on taking a selfie every single time she visits my office. It's become our tradition. She pulls out her phone, grins wide, and says, "Say cheese, Doc."

At first, I wondered if it blurred the lines of professionalism. But over time, I realized what it really did: it turned the sterile ritual of a medical visit into something personal, something joyful. In those moments, she isn't just my patient and I'm not just her doctor — we're two people sharing a laugh, marking a moment, building trust one snapshot at a time.

Those photos live in her camera roll, not her chart. But to her, they're part of her care. They remind her that medicine isn't only about lab results or prescriptions — it's about feeling seen, feeling valued, and knowing she matters. And for me, they're a reminder too: that sometimes the smallest traditions, even a quick selfie, can carry the most meaning.

When her mother passed away, it was devastating. Since then, this patient has weathered her own health challenges, yet when she walks into my outpatient clinic with her daughter by her side, there's joy on her face. She's genuinely happy to be there. Happy to see me. She doesn't dread her appointment; she looks forward to it.

I've known her for years. I cared for the woman she called "Mom," a woman she loved deeply. Some might call this unprofessional. A violation of the sacred doctor-patient boundary. I don't see it that way. I see a human being who trusts me — deeply. I see a long-standing relationship that's grown beyond the exam room, rooted in mutual respect and care. I see a moment of gratitude. A snapshot of connection.

She thinks I'm wonderful. She says so publicly. She posts our selfies to social media. She writes about how lucky she is to have me as her doctor. And you know what? I feel lucky to have her as my patient. She's one of my biggest supporters, and I'm proud to be part of her story.

Not long ago, she arrived for her appointment and realized she'd forgotten her phone. She looked genuinely disappointed — not because she couldn't check her messages, but because she couldn't get our much-needed photo.

So I reached into my pocket, pulled out my phone, and said, "Let's take one on mine." I snapped the picture. Then I asked gently, "Would it be okay if I shared this one too?"

She laughed. Of course it was. In fact, she told me she wanted me to. For her, it wasn't just about a picture; it was about being seen, about celebrating the simple joy of connection in a space where most people expect only seriousness.

In that moment, I realized something important: The selfie wasn't about breaking boundaries. It was about strengthening them — about building a bridge between doctor and patient, one smile at a time.

That photo doesn't weaken the doctor-patient bond. It strengthens it. It turns the visit into more than numbers and lab results. It reminds the patient that she matters not just as a case, but as a person. And if that looks unconventional to some, so be it. Medicine is not a performance of detachment. It's a practice of presence. And sometimes, presence looks like leaning into a moment of joy and saying, "Cheese."

On the Matter of Professionalism

Why is a doctor posting selfies with patients? Isn't that crossing a line? Isn't that a little...unprofessional?

Let's talk about boundaries.

Yes, there is a line between being a doctor and being a friend. Boundaries matter. They protect both patients and physicians. But that line doesn't mean we have to be distant. It doesn't mean we can't care personally. It doesn't mean we can't celebrate the relationships we've built with the very people who trust us with their lives.

Because medicine isn't only about treating illness. It's about showing up fully human in the exam room — willing to share in laughter as well as tears, in small traditions as well as serious conversations.

Connection doesn't compromise professionalism. Connection is professionalism — because healing starts not with detachment, but with trust. I'm a doctor, but I'm a human being first. She's my patient. But she's a human being too. There's no power dynamic here. No hidden agenda. She doesn't expect anything beyond what I already give: my full attention, my medical judgment, my time, my respect. And I don't expect anything from her, either — except for her trust.

She brings me little gifts sometimes. Trinkets she's found. Antiques she knows I'll appreciate. Is that crossing the line too? I don't think so. That's called connection. That's the product of years of consistency and compassion, not impropriety.

We have a relationship built on openness and kindness. She knows about my family. She has commented on my wife's Instagram photos, complimented our kids, cheered us on. Is that unprofessional? Or is that what it looks like when a patient sees her doctor as a whole person — and is seen as one in return?

We talk a lot in medicine about burnout. About disconnection. About the isolation physicians feel in a system that prioritizes volume over value. And yet when a patient dares to care for her doctor, we raise concerns about "professionalism."

I think we've misunderstood the point. This woman doesn't take a selfie with me because she wants attention. She does it because she wants to remember the person who's helped her through some of the most difficult moments of her life. She wants to capture that sense of safety, of continuity, of gratitude.

I don't need to tell her, "Let's keep this focused on your health." She knows why she's here. She shows up. She takes her medications. She follows up. Yet she also brings joy into the room — and leaves a little behind for me, too.

This idea that doctors must remain emotionally distant in order to be effective? That's outdated. It's a relic of a time when vulnerability was mistaken for weakness, when detachment was confused with professionalism.

I don't practice that way. And I don't want to. Because distance doesn't heal; it isolates. Patients don't need a wall; they need a witness. They need a doctor who can hold space for both the science and the humanity of what they're going through.

Vulnerability isn't a liability; it's a bridge. It's what allows us to meet patients where they are, to connect beyond the lab results and the exam table, to show them they are not alone. So no, I don't believe that caring deeply makes me less effective. I believe it makes me better. It keeps me human in a profession that too often demands we act otherwise.

What about precedent? What about the next patient?

I've been asked whether allowing one patient to take selfies sets a precedent. Would every patient start expecting the same? Would it blur the line until there was no line left? The thought lingered. The worry about setting a standard I couldn't maintain. The fear of a boundary crossed.

But here's what I realized: Precedent isn't the same as permission. Not every patient wants the same thing, and not every relationship looks the same. What matters is intention and context.

For this patient, the selfie isn't about crossing boundaries. It's about honoring the relationship, celebrating her resilience, and bringing joy into a space that often feels heavy. For another patient, that might look different: a handshake, a shared laugh, a few extra minutes of listening.

Professionalism doesn't mean treating every patient the exact same way. It means showing up with the same respect, the same care, the same commitment to boundaries — while recognizing that human connection doesn't come in a single form.

So, I'm not afraid of precedent. Each patient is different. Every relationship is different. What matters is intention. If a photo strengthens a patient's sense of agency, trust, or joy, why should I resist that?

Some will say, "This makes me uneasy. What if it gets taken out of context?" And I understand that concern. But context is everything. And in this context, the relationship is healthy, respectful, and deeply human. That's all I need to know. Because medicine is not about appearances; it's about presence. It's not about how the outside world interprets a moment, but how the patient experiences it.

If a simple photo builds trust, if it brings joy into a room that too often carries fear, then that is not a breach of professionalism. It's the heart of it.

I'm not blind to the risks. Consent matters. Privacy matters. I've taken care to protect both. I've thought carefully about what I share, how I share it, and why. But I refuse to let fear dictate how I show up for my patients — especially when they show up fully for me.

Trust is a two-way street. If a patient invites me into their life with openness and joy, then honoring that moment with respect is not a breach of professionalism; it's an extension of it.

Caution has its place, but so does connection. And in medicine, the moments that endure are not only the charts we complete or the labs we order — they're the moments when we allow ourselves to be human, together.

Maybe your practice is different. Maybe your comfort level is different. Yet don't mistake connection for impropriety. Don't assume that friendship negates professionalism. To me, this isn't a boundary violation; it's a boundary redefinition — that makes space for empathy, joy, and humanity.

And I'm honored to be in it.

PART II

Inside the Exam Room

Enter the crucible of residency: the sleepless nights, the fluorescent hallways, the relentless demand to prove you belong. Here, medicine tests spirit as much as skill. I learned that residency was not just about treating patients; it was about facing myself. Medicine was never about answers; it was about showing up, again and again, until it became who I was.

BECOMING A DOCTOR IS ONE THING; being one day after day, patient after patient is something else entirely. Inside the exam room, the science of medicine collides with the weight of human emotion. These are the moments that define our practice — not diagnoses and treatments, but connection, vulnerability, and the courage to show up with your full self. The moments that define outpatient clinical medicine beyond textbooks and diagnoses.

Being a doctor is about more than diagnosing illnesses or prescribing medications. It's about more than knowing the latest research, the right drug dose, or the most effective treatment plan. Of course those things matter, but they're part of the job description.

Imagine what it's like to sit in the waiting room before your appointment. You're holding onto questions you've been rehearsing in your head for weeks, maybe months. You're worried about the test result that came back "abnormal." You're nervous to talk about the chest discomfort you've been ignoring. You're carrying the weight of something you haven't told anyone — not even your spouse — and now you're about to walk into an exam room and lay it all on the table for someone you may barely know.

That's a lot to ask of anyone.

In every encounter, I try to remember what it feels like to be on the other side of the desk, and that's why I endeavor to make the relationship personal from the beginning. It's not about making small talk. It's about building trust.

When someone trusts you, they will open up. They will tell you the details you need to make the right decisions for their health. They will trust your recommendations, even when the news isn't what they hoped for. And they will feel seen — not as a case, not as a diagnosis, but as a person.

I believe the first 30 seconds of any patient interaction can make or break the connection. It starts the moment I walk through the door.

If I'm smiling, relaxed, and genuinely happy to see them, it shows. If I greet them by name and recall something they told me last visit — maybe how their daughter's wedding went or how they've been adjusting to retirement — they know I've been paying attention.

If I rush in with my eyes glued to the computer screen, firing off questions without looking up, the opportunity to build trust slips away. Patients can sense when you're going through the motions. They know when they're a chart instead of a person.

So I slow down. I remind myself: Medicine isn't just about data collection — it's about presence.

If they're nervous, I acknowledge it. A simple, "I know this feels overwhelming, but you're not alone in it," can change the room. If they're in pain, I validate it before launching into the next step. Sometimes the most important treatment is simply saying, "I hear you." If they're worried, I listen before I speak. The silence might stretch, but often what fills it is the truth they've been holding back. If they're closed off, I look for a crack in the wall — humor, kindness, patience. Whatever it takes to remind them I see more than their symptoms.

Connection doesn't happen by accident; it happens in the pauses, the acknowledgments, the human gestures that remind patients they matter. Sometimes that connection happens in seconds; sometimes it takes the entire visit. If you get it right in the beginning, the rest of the encounter becomes easier for both of you.

In primary care, these relationships can span years, even decades. I've been the first person they've called with good news and the one they've turned to in moments of devastation. Still, connection isn't only for long-term relationships. Even in specialties where you might see a patient once or twice, the opportunity is still there. You may not walk with them for years, but you can leave an impression that lasts. You can be the doctor they remember — not for how quickly you diagnosed their condition, but for how you made them feel: The one who listened. The one who explained things clearly. The one who treated them like a person instead of a chart.

Patients don't always remember every detail of what we prescribe or explain. But they never forget how we showed up for them at the moment they needed us most. I've had patients tell me, "You're the first doctor who's ever explained it to me in a way I could understand." That always stops me in my tracks. For that's not about intelligence — it's about communication.

Honesty matters in medicine. But honesty without clarity? It can sound like a foreign language. So I try to explain things in a way that is not only accurate, but relatable. I reach for metaphors, for plain words, for examples that connect medicine to daily life. Because what good is the truth if it gets lost in translation?

If a patient can walk out of the room and explain their condition to a friend in plain language, then I know I've done my job. Because real communication isn't about proving how much I know; it's about making sure my patient feels informed, empowered, and understood.

Patients come to us with high expectations — and rightly so. When they walk into my office, they are trusting me with their health, their future. And sometimes even their life. They expect me to have the answers — or at least to find them. That expectation is harder to measure, but it's every bit as important as prescribing the right medication or ordering the correct test.

It's why a patient will follow through with a treatment plan — or why they won't. It's why they'll be honest about their symptoms — or why they'll hold back. It's why they'll trust your judgment — or quietly second-guess everything you say.

We track blood pressure, lab values, and imaging results with precision. But we don't chart the nod of reassurance, the careful explanation, or the silence we hold while a patient finds the words they've been afraid to say. And yet, those moments often determine whether the science we offer actually takes root. The medicine only works if the relationship does too.

The Two-Way Mirror

The trust between a doctor and a patient isn't built on outpatient clinical knowledge alone. It's built on a sense of safety, respect, and genuine connection.

One of the things I have come to understand over the years is that patients are observing us as much as we're observing them. They notice how we walk into the room — whether we stand tall or slump from exhaustion. They notice if we make eye contact or keep glancing at the clock. They notice if our tone is warm or flat.

We're trained to take in every detail about our patients — their expressions, their posture, their choice of words — but we sometimes forget they're doing the same with us. That means every visit is a two-way mirror. I'm assessing them, but they're also deciding — sometimes in seconds — whether they can trust me, whether I'm listening, whether I'm worth opening up to.

I'll never forget one patient who came in for what seemed like a routine visit. She was quiet, polite, and gave short answers to my questions. Her blood pressure was fine. Her labs from last month were normal. On paper, she was healthy.

Still, something didn't feel right. Instead of moving on to my next patient, I paused. I asked how she was really doing.

Her eyes welled up. She told me she had recently lost her husband and had been feeling completely alone. She hadn't planned on bringing it up — it wasn't on her "list" for the visit. But she admitted, almost in a whisper, that she didn't know who else to talk to.

So we set aside the lab results and the checklist. We spent most of the appointment talking about grief, loneliness, and support systems. I connected her with a counselor and encouraged her to reach out to a neighbor she'd mentioned in passing — someone who had once brought her dinner after the funeral.

A few months later, she returned. This time her face carried more light. She told me that conversation had been a turning point. It hadn't erased the grief, but it had reminded her she wasn't as alone as she thought.

Moments like that never show up in the chart. There's no billing code for presence. But that doesn't make it any less essential. Sometimes the most powerful medicine we offer is simply the space to be heard.

That experience reminded me that sometimes the most important thing you can do as a doctor has nothing to do with a prescription pad. Sometimes it's noticing what's unsaid. Each patient encounter is an opportunity to set the bar for what a medical relationship should look like. For me, that means walking in with presence — the act of being wholly there, listening without rushing, being honest without being cold, and making sure my patients know I'm on their side.

It also means remembering that we are human, too. We have our own worries, our own fatigue, our own challenges outside of work. Yet when I step into that exam room, my role is clear. My patient deserves my attention, my expertise, and my compassion — no matter what's going on in my own life.

Medicine will always be about science, evidence, and skill. Yet the truth in medicine — the part that patients remember long after the visit — is the human connection. It's the smile, the pause, the willingness to sit in someone's discomfort with them. It's the ability to see beyond the chart to the person sitting in front of you.

For in the end, the best care doesn't come from knowing the medicine. It comes from knowing the patient.

A Day in the Life

Most mornings start with a wake-up call — sometimes literal; sometimes internal. I try to begin the day with a workout. The gym is down the road, and I like to get there early. Sometimes I'm the first one in. It's quiet. Peaceful. A moment for myself before the storm begins.

What do I mean by that? In a life where I pour so much into others, these quiet moments are how I breathe.

Clinic life is full — often overwhelming. I manage a large panel of patients and a schedule that rarely has breathing room. I get to the office early, already anticipating what awaits: a full inbox, lab results to review, consult notes, refill requests, and patient messages — always more patient messages, every day. I used to dread it. Now, I accept it. I chose this life. I choose to be busy.

My two medical assistants are already at work when I arrive, sifting through the digital chaos to bring order to the day. We try not to stare at the schedule for too long. It's like looking up at a mountain you're about to climb: dozens of patients, dozens of needs, dozens of decisions.

The day officially starts at 8:30 a.m. Once it begins, it doesn't stop. I do my best to see each patient who needs to be seen and answer each question that comes my way. Maybe I overextend myself. Maybe I'm too accommodating. That's debatable. Yet I'd rather be the doctor who goes out of his way than the one who turns patients away because he's "too busy."

There's barely time for a drink of water, let alone lunch. Sometimes I jot a note between rooms, reply to a message in a spare moment. Juggling in-person visits and electronic communication is an art form — triage in real time.

As I enter each room, I remind myself: I must be the same doctor. No matter what emotion I carried from the last encounter, I leave it at the door. That's one of the hardest parts of medicine: compartmentalizing. In one room, you hear an uplifting story. In the next, a devastating one. You absorb pain, deliver hope, hold uncertainty — and then pivot. Quietly. Seamlessly.

Even when I am not feeling my best, I do my best to act like I am. Because patients don't just see the white coat; they feel the energy that comes with it. If I carry exhaustion, frustration, or doubt into the room, it lingers. It colors the encounter.

So I steady myself. I breathe. I remind myself that for the person sitting across from me, this visit might be the most important part of their week. They deserve my full attention, even if I'm running on fumes.

It's not about pretending I'm invincible; it's about offering steadiness when their world feels unsteady. And in doing that I sometimes find strength I didn't know I had.

I take a "lunch break," though it's rarely that. Maybe a protein bar, some water, a cup of tea if I'm lucky. More often it's a quick scroll through morning charts, a handful of lab results, a few patient messages that can't wait.

It's not really rest — it's a pause, a breath.

Because the truth is, medicine doesn't stop at noon. The work keeps moving, and so do we. And in those few minutes, I try to gather myself — not just to keep going, but to show up for the next patient as if they're the first.

By 1:00 p.m., the afternoon rush begins. The schedule is packed — sometimes double-booked. I do that on purpose. My patients want to see me — not urgent care, not a covering provider. They trust me. That trust is sacred, and I owe them my time. Not every doctor agrees with this approach. That's okay, because in the end, this is my practice, my choice, my way.

Mid-afternoon, the sick calls start piling up, We adapt. We shift. We accommodate. My team is tireless in keeping the day moving. I never take for granted that I'm lucky to work with them.

By 4:00 p.m., the waiting room begins to quiet. From the outside, it looks like the day is winding down, yet this is when another shift begins. Lab reviews. Documentation. Messages. Refills. Notes. All the things I couldn't do between patients, I do now.

That's the soundtrack of modern medicine: more clicks than conversations. The work doesn't end when the last patient leaves. There are charts to finish, codes to enter, boxes to check. Entire evenings lost — not to thinking about patients, but to documenting them.

Some days it feels like medicine today isn't about caring; it's about compliance. It's not about presence; it's about paperwork. It's not about listening; it's about liability.

And yet, every box I check pulls me further from the reason I went into medicine in the first place. The system demands documentation, but patients demand connection. And the truth is, you can't serve both fully at the same time. That's the paradox we live in: To prove we care, we spend less time actually caring.

By 5:00 p.m., I aim to finish. I want to get home to my family. They deserve my presence too. Eventually, the inbox is clean. The charts are closed. The adrenaline fades. That tingly feeling? That's me returning to myself. Tomorrow, I'll do it all again.

This is the life I chose, and the truth is that I love it. I love the pace. I love the connection. I love the privilege of being someone's doctor. And even when it's hard, I'm grateful.

Seeing and Being Seen

What patients long for isn't just someone to listen with their ears, but someone to listen with their presence: Someone who notices when a voice cracks or when shoulders slump. Someone who recognizes that silence can be as telling as words. Someone who sees not a collection of symptoms, but a whole person: fragile, complicated, resilient, trying to make sense of what life has handed them.

Because true listening isn't passive. It's active, deliberate, embodied. It says: I see you, I hear you, you matter. And sometimes, that's the most powerful medicine we can offer.

This need is not unique; it's deeply human. Some people live solitary lives and are content with it. But more often, I find the opposite: patients who crave connection, who yearn for someone to talk to, to lean on, to simply be there. They don't just want a physician; they want a partner, a companion, a steady presence in a world that often feels unsteady. They want someone who will look after them not only medically, but emotionally; someone who will call them by name, remember the stories they shared last visit, and recognize the small details that make them who they are.

Because for many patients, healing doesn't begin with prescriptions or lab results. It begins with presence, with knowing they matter enough to be remembered.

Sure, there are people who prefer to be alone. I have patients who live quiet lives, who value solitude, who are content in their own company. For them, independence is its own kind of strength, and they don't always want — or need — someone to fill the silence.

But even then, I've learned that solitude doesn't mean the absence of connection. It just means the connection looks different. Sometimes it's a brief conversation, a small gesture of recognition, or the reassurance that someone is paying attention. Even the most independent patients want to know they're seen.

That's what medicine is about. At least, that's what I believe it should be about.

We aren't just physicians. For many people, we are the only steady presence they have in their lives. Not just someone to manage blood pressure or refill prescriptions, but someone to count on. Someone to call. Someone who cares enough to show up again and again.

Because when the clinic doors close and the charts are filed away, what stays with patients isn't only the treatment plan — it's the reassurance that they weren't facing it alone. And maybe that's the quiet truth of this profession: At its best, medicine is less about curing disease and more about reminding people they still matter.

Over the years, I've had many patients rely on me for more than a diagnosis. I've been asked to be an emergency contact, a decision-maker, a surrogate family member. One patient once told me, only half-joking, "I trust you more than I trust my husband." To be fair, it wasn't her first marriage, but still, the sentiment was genuine. What does it say about our world, about our support systems, when a patient feels closer to their physician than to anyone else in their life? It says something profound — and heartbreaking — about loneliness.

I used to be surprised by how many of my patients lacked close family or social support. Now, I'm no longer surprised, yet I am deeply affected.

Loneliness is one of the quietest epidemics in healthcare. You won't find it coded on the problem list. It doesn't show up in a lab result or a radiology report, yet its effects are everywhere.

It shows up in subtle ways: missed appointments, worsening chronic conditions, increased ER visits, vague symptoms that don't fit cleanly into any diagnosis. And it shows up emotionally: in the long silences between questions, in the sigh before someone says, "I'm fine," in the way a patient lingers at the end of the visit, not quite ready to leave.

For many, I'm the only person they'll speak to all week. That's a humbling responsibility — and a heavy one.

For many of my older patients, the senior center is more than just a building; it's a heartbeat of community. It's where friendships are kept alive, where laughter is shared over coffee, and where small celebrations carry the weight of holidays. For some, it's the only place they feel truly seen.

That's why I always ask about it. It's become part of our ritual. "What are you doing today?" "Any trips coming up?"

Their faces light up as they tell me about bingo nights, exercise classes, or the occasional bus trip. Sometimes I'll hear about a holiday party, or who brought the best casserole to the potluck. They even have a homecoming each year, complete with a homecoming queen crowned in front of the entire group.

For many, the senior center isn't just a way to pass the time. It's a lifeline, a reminder that they belong, that their stories and presence still matter. Many are widowed; this is their fight against loneliness. And when they share those stories with me, it's more than small talk; it's part of their health. Loneliness weighs heavily; connection heals in ways no prescription can.

Every so often, I hear I've even become the talk of the day. Going to see me is treated like an event, something to brag about: "I saw my doctor today." They'll say it proudly, as though it's a story worth sharing with friends. And in a way, it is. Because it means the visit wasn't just about blood pressure readings or medication adjustments — it was about being seen, cared for, and valued.

Those conversations about bingo and bus trips may never show up in the chart. There's no billing code for "asked about homecoming queen." But they matter. They remind me and my patients that medicine is more than treatment. It's relationship. And sometimes, a minute spent talking about the senior center does more good than anything I could prescribe.

We talk a lot in medicine about the burden of documentation, the frustrations of prior authorizations, the inefficiencies of the electronic health record, yet the emotional weight of bearing witness to another person's isolation rarely makes it into the conversation. Yet it's one of the most sacred and difficult parts of this job.

Loneliness doesn't erode the spirit. It takes a toll on the body. It contributes to depression, anxiety, cognitive decline. And even early death. Studies have shown that chronic loneliness can be as harmful to health as smoking 15 cigarettes a day. That's not poetic exaggeration; that's outpatient clinical evidence.

I see it in young adults — especially those who are navigating illness alone — who feel unseen in a world so loud with curated images of happiness and belonging. I see it in middle-aged patients who never married, who devoted themselves to careers or caretaking, and now find themselves quietly adrift. Loneliness doesn't discriminate; it's a slow, smoldering burn, a quiet ache that builds until it becomes unbearable. It's that pit in your stomach, the anxious energy that doesn't go away, the desperate desire to be needed, to be missed, to be noticed. It's not sadness; it's a loss of orientation, a sense that no one would even know if you disappeared.

As physicians, we're given a remarkable opportunity to be the interruption in that narrative, the person who does notice, who does care, who does call back.

No, we can't solve loneliness with a stethoscope, but we can acknowledge it. We can name it for what it is, instead of pretending it doesn't exist. We can meet it with kindness, with patience, with presence. And sometimes, that's enough to soften the edges of grief, enough to change the course of a day, and occasionally, enough to change the course of a life.

Because medicine isn't always about cures; often, it's about connection. And in a world that leaves so many people feeling unseen, even the smallest gesture of presence can be the most powerful medicine we offer.

I have come to understand that healing doesn't always come in the form of a pill. Sometimes, healing is in the way we sit, the way we listen, the way we remember details from last visit, the way we say "I'm glad you're here" and mean it.

A senior walking club. A church group. A book club. A fitness class. Sometimes, it takes a few tries, yet when they find something that clicks — when they start telling me stories about new friends or a community that gives them joy — it's like watching a light turn on.

Of course, we also have to offer tangible guidance. When I suspect loneliness is contributing to depression, I talk to my patients about joining a local group or center. Going from loneliness to belonging isn't emotional — it's physiologic. It breathes life back into people. It restores appetite, sleep, motivation. It gives people a reason to take care of themselves again.

And watching that happen? It's one of the greatest rewards in medicine.

No, I can't be everything to each patient. I'm not their family. I'm not their therapist. I'm not their savior. Yet I am someone who sees them. And sometimes, that's more than enough. When we show up for people — especially those who feel like no one else will — we remind them they're not invisible. We remind them that they matter.

So I'll continue to be more than a doctor. I'll be a witness, a supporter, a presence. Sometimes, what patients need most isn't a diagnosis. I'm honored to be that someone.

Reflections on Death

One of the most common questions people outside medicine ask me is this: How do you deal with death?

They usually ask with a mix of curiosity and hesitation, as if the words themselves might be too heavy to say out loud. People wonder how we can sit at the bedside of someone who is slipping away, or how we can walk into a room knowing that nothing we prescribe will change the outcome.

The truth is, there's no simple answer. You don't "deal" with death; you live alongside it. You carry it with you. Sometimes it's quiet acceptance. Sometimes it's gut-wrenching grief. And sometimes it's the strange, sacred privilege of holding space for a family's last moments together.

Death never becomes routine; it never stops mattering. But you learn to make peace with its presence, because without that acceptance, you couldn't go on.

And maybe that's the real answer: You don't deal with death by shutting it out. You deal with it by showing up anyway, by standing in the room when it would be easier to walk away, by remembering that even in the final chapter, there's still room for compassion, dignity, and presence.

When a hospice notice arrives, I know what it means: the beginning of the end. And I feel it deeply. I've poured myself into this person — my heart, my drive, my passion. I've sat with them in their struggle, adjusted medications, tried every path forward. I've watched them fight, decline, rally, and fight again. And then, one day, the notice appears in my inbox or on my desk.

It's only a piece of paper, but it feels heavier than that. Because shortly after it comes, I know it won't be long before the next message arrives — the one that tells me they've passed away. Every time, I pause. I think of their face, their family, the journey we've walked together. It's not just a patient file closing; it's a relationship ending. A thread of connection cut. And while part of me braces for it, another part refuses to grow numb. Because if I ever stop feeling that weight, if those notices ever become just paperwork, then I've lost something essential.

The question of how I deal with death? People don't mean it philosophically. They mean it in the most human, intimate sense: How do you manage losing someone you've taken care of for years? How do you carry on when a patient — someone you've fought to keep alive — dies?

It's not about theory. It's about the chair left empty in the exam room, the voice you'll never hear again, the family who walks in carrying only memory. It's about the weight of absence and what it takes to keep showing up anyway.

It's an interesting question, and not an easy one. I've become familiar with its timing, although the truth is, it often makes no sense at all.

Some people die young, with no warning, no family history, no obvious risk factors. Others beat the odds for decades. Some chain-smoke into their 90s. Others live clean and still die young.

Medicine humbles you into recognizing that life rarely follows the rules we expect. It teaches us that health and longevity are never guaranteed, that the line between living and dying can be razor-thin. And in the end, it leaves you with this: an appreciation for just how fragile — and how arbitrary — life can be. I wouldn't say we become numb to it, yet we do become used to it. We get familiar with death's unpredictability.

There's no single answer to the question of why someone dies — no tidy algorithm — and maybe that's what's hardest for people to understand. They want explanations and so do we. Yet death resists logic; it resists fairness. Still, it's part of our world — constant undercurrent.

They become part of us — a different kind of family. Over the years, I carry the truth of their lives with me: their kids' names, their jobs, their favorite foods, their quirks. I've watched them grow older, weather illnesses, celebrate milestones. Maybe I don't know everything, but I know enough — enough to feel like, in some way, we belong to each other.

Patients are not "cases." They're not boxes to chart and check off. They are people whose stories have intertwined with ours, whose presence lingers long after the appointment ends. That is the privilege of continuity: To watch lives unfold not in snapshots, but in chapters. To carry not just their diagnoses, but their humanity. And in doing so, to be reminded of our own.

So when one of them dies, the first thing I want to know is: What happened? Even when I'm the one who fills out the death certificate, I find myself digging through the record. Trying to make sense of it. It's not a chart anymore; it's a story that ended. I want to know the final chapter.

Sometimes it hurts to read those notes, knowing this person I knew for years is gone, that I'll never see their name on my schedule again, that their spouse, who is also my patient, will now be sitting in my office alone.

In those moments, I have to hold space for both my own grief and theirs. I might walk into the exam room and learn, without warning, that someone's husband died two days ago. Maybe it was sudden; maybe it was expected. Either way, I have to respond — to be a doctor, but also a human, to offer empathy and composure, to bear witness and guide them through the fog.

This is one of the quiet burdens of being a physician. We don't take care of people while they're alive. We carry them after they're gone and somehow, we learn to move forward.

One of the skills I've come to rely on most is the ability to compartmentalize. It's not emotional avoidance or apathy; it's survival. Compartmentalizing allows me to function — not as a doctor, but as a human being. It's what helps me walk into that exam room, stay present, listen deeply, and respond with care without breaking down in the moment. It lets me hold space for someone else's grief without being swallowed by my own.

I have come to understand how to separate parts of myself — at least temporarily. My thoughts, emotions, and personal reactions.

When I'm in the room with a patient whose entire world has just changed, I can't let my own response take center stage, so I set it aside. It's not ignored — just shelved, held for a quieter time, when I'm not the one being leaned on, when I'm not the one who needs to carry the weight of someone else's grief or fear.

It doesn't mean I don't feel it; it means I make space for the patient first. And later — sometimes much later — I return to those emotions, take them down from the shelf, and allow myself to process them in my own way.

Because to practice medicine is not to be unfeeling; it's to feel deeply, but also to know when those feelings belong in the room and when they must wait. This mental discipline doesn't make me cold; it makes me capable. It gives me room to be a physician in moments that demand stability, when a family looks to me for clarity and strength. And it gives me room to be a father, a husband, a friend without bringing the full weight of loss into every corner of my life.

The grief is still there. The emotions are real. But by placing them where they belong, I can keep showing up for my patients and for the people I love. That balance isn't detachment; it's survival. And it's what allows me to keep practicing medicine with both presence and humanity.

In many ways, compartmentalization is the unspoken lifeline of medical practice. It's the boundary we set so we can stay soft without falling apart. It's the pause button we press to protect our own mental health.

Of course, the grief finds us. The sadness catches up. Yet when we give ourselves permission to feel it on our own terms, we can show up better for those who need us: our patients, their families, and our own.

We often think of medicine as a science of healing. Yet sometimes, the truest healing comes in knowing when to hold space and when to set it aside.

You don't get used to death. You get better at carrying it.

The Importance of Silence

In the outpatient clinical world, silence can say everything that words fail to express. And yet, as physicians, we're trained to speak — to explain, to reassure, to fill the space with answers.

But what happens when the right words don't come? Or worse, when words aren't what's needed at all?

Sometimes the greatest act of care isn't speaking, but sitting in the silence, bearing witness without trying to fix, holding space when there are no easy explanations or solutions. Because silence, when it's shared, isn't empty; it's presence. And in the right moment, presence can heal in ways language never could.

I've come to learn that silence is not the absence of communication; it is a form of it — one that's often louder, more profound, and more emotionally charged than the longest monologue.

There have been times when a patient finished telling me something deeply personal — a diagnosis they're processing, a fear they haven't shared with anyone else, a grief that doesn't have neat edges — and then nothing. No follow-up question, no words to fill the space. Just quiet. The younger version of myself might have rushed to respond. I might have filled that silence with medical terms, reassurances, or a pivot to the next step. Yet now, with more years in practice — and more mistakes behind me — I've come to understand that silence deserves its own kind of reverence.

When a patient falls silent, they are not always done speaking; they are gathering themselves. They are letting what was said settle into the space between us. My job isn't to interrupt that process; it's to honor it.

Sometimes silence is uncomfortable, awkward, heavy. You can feel the tension settle into the room — the weight of unspoken questions. And in those moments, both sides are wondering: Should I say something? Are they waiting for me to speak? Are they finished? Am I being too quiet? Too abrupt? Too cold?

The air thickens with uncertainty, and the instinct — mine, theirs — is to fill it. To rescue the moment with words. But I've learned that if I can hold steady, if I can resist the urge to smooth over the silence, something often happens.

The pause becomes permission. The space becomes invitation. The silence becomes the opening for truths that might never surface otherwise.

Because silence isn't absence. It's presence, stretched out long enough for someone to gather courage and speak what they're carrying. Silence isn't absence. It's invitation. That's where presence — the act of being wholly there — matters most.

True communication is about more than words; it's about timing, attention, and empathy. It's about noticing the raised eyebrow, the shift in posture, the sigh that speaks louder than a sentence. It's about understanding that people from different cultures, backgrounds, and personalities relate to silence in different ways. For some, silence is respect; for others, it feels unsettling, even cold.

The work, then, is not to impose my own comfort level, but to read the room, to know when silence is an invitation — and when it's a burden. To let the patient's needs — not my unease — shape the moment. Because at its best, silence isn't emptiness; it's presence. And presence, when offered with empathy, is its own kind of language. That's what makes medicine such a human art.

I once had a patient — a woman in her late 70s — who came in for what should have been a routine visit. Vitals stable. Medications unchanged. Labs normal. And yet, something was off. Her posture was heavy. Her eyes wouldn't meet mine. Her hands fidgeted with the edge of her scarf.

I asked how she was. She answered, "Fine." And then silence. I didn't rush. I didn't change the subject. I waited. Eventually, in a voice barely above a whisper, she said, "My husband passed last month."

That pause, that silence — it had been her opening. Her way of saying, "Please notice something's not right." If I had hurried past it, I would have missed the truth. Moments like that remind me that silence is not empty. It is full. It can carry grief. It can carry fear. It can even carry hope. You just have to be patient enough to hear it.

Silence also plays a role in joy, in awe, in connection. The quiet after a parent hears that their child's scan is clear. The breath held when you say, "It's benign." The stillness after the laughter fades but the feeling lingers.

Not all silence is heavy; some of it is sacred.

In our fast-moving world, silence is often mistaken for emptiness. Yet in medicine, we know better. We must. Because silence isn't nothing — it's everything left unsaid. It's the pause where relief settles in, where fear releases its grip, where hope quietly takes root. Learning to hold silence — truly hold it — is part of what makes a doctor trusted. It's part of what builds the relationship. Not the scripts. Not the protocols. The pause. The space. The presence.

It's not easy.

Still sometimes, doing something means doing nothing. It means listening, waiting, being. And that doesn't come naturally. It takes practice. It takes confidence — not in your knowledge, but in your humility. It takes emotional intelligence and a willingness to be uncomfortable in the service of someone else's process.

As a doctor, you're not treating bodies; you're engaging with souls, and souls don't always speak in words. So yes, silence can be deafening. It's in the silence that we see what's going on. It's in the silence that we invite someone to be seen. It's in the silence that we learn to be present — not as physicians, but as people.

Making Me Who I Am

I don't have one patient who shaped me. Instead, I have hundreds — each one leaving a trace, each encounter adding another layer to who I've become. I've been molded gradually, over time, by the accumulation of everyday moments. Some were profound, others barely perceptible in the moment. Yet together, they've changed me.

They ask about my kids by name, remember their ages, want to know how school is going, what sports they're playing, what they're up to this summer. Some of these patients have been with me since I started this practice more than a decade ago.

When I was still finding my rhythm as a young attending, they offered me grace. When I became a father, they offered me advice. Over time, many of them have come to treat me like their own son. Some don't have children of their own. For them, I am the closest thing they have. And in that role, I've come to understand that medicine is more than clinical care; it's companionship, continuity, and presence woven into the fabric of someone's life.

Medicine isn't just about me shaping their lives — it's about them shaping mine. Over the years, my patients have taught me patience, humility, and perspective. They've taught me that medicine is not a one-way street, but a relationship that deepens with time. And that, perhaps more than anything else, has made me the doctor I am today.

One patient brought me a framed quote she said reminded her of me. Another handed me two old medical books on general surgery, their covers worn, their pages faded with age. They weren't just antiques; the books had been passed down from her father, who was a surgeon in the late 1800s. To anyone else, they might have looked like relics for a shelf. But to her, they were a piece of family history, a link to her father's life's work. Placing them in my hands wasn't about giving me objects — it was about entrusting me with something sacred, a gesture of faith that I would honor the same calling he once carried.

Over the years, the gifts have been just as varied as the patients who gave them. I now have a binder of old cigarette cards — something I didn't even know existed until a patient handed them to me. Each card is set carefully into position, like a binder of collectible baseball cards. To him, they weren't just cards; they were memories, pieces of a hobby he loved, a slice of his own story. And in giving them to me, he wasn't offering me cardboard rectangles — he was offering me a piece of himself.

These gestures aren't transactional; they rarely have any nominal value. Most of the gifts I've received would mean little to anyone outside the relationship. But to the people offering them, they mean everything, and because of that, they mean everything to me.

A bookmark tucked into a card. A recipe written on a slip of paper. A photo from a family vacation. A scarf, knitted slowly by hands stiff with arthritis. None of these would sell at an auction, but each carries something no market can measure: thought, intention, memory, connection.

They speak to a relationship that transcends the exam room. They remind me that being someone's doctor isn't just about managing blood pressure or adjusting medications — it's about being invited into the fabric of someone's life.

And then there are the handwritten notes. Not quick thank-yous, but deeply personal letters — recollections, affirmations, reflections. Stories of how our time together mattered in ways I could never have captured in a chart.

These are the gifts that stay with me. They don't sit on a shelf so much as they live in my heart. They remind me that the doctor–patient relationship is never one-directional. It's reciprocal. And sometimes, the most valuable gifts I'm given aren't objects at all, but reminders of the profound privilege it is to be trusted with someone's life and story.

The calm and the chaotic. The nice and the mad. Primary care doesn't shield you from anything — it exposes you to everything. People don't bring their blood pressure readings or lab results. They bring their whole selves, their fears, their frustrations, their stories. And if you're listening, you begin to see that the job is less about fixing and more about witnessing. Holding space. Walking with people, not ahead of them.

I've been shaped by the good and the bad, the joyful and the grieving. I've had patients with dementia who can't remember their own address but somehow remember my name. Some of the patients who've shaped me most are the ones I've seen decline. I've watched them transition from driving themselves to visits, to arriving with caregivers, to moving into assisted living, and finally to hospice.

I try to listen. I try to show up. I try to do right by them. There's something about continuity — about trust built slowly, visit by visit — that becomes a bond neither diagnosis nor distance can undo.

Sometimes it's something small: adjusting a medication to ease a side effect. Sometimes it's a simple follow-up: "Feeling a bit better today — thank you for listening last week." What I've learned is that patients don't always want a cure; more often, they want to feel heard, feel known. And for some, this relationship — the rhythm of mutual respect, the constancy of presence — becomes more than healthcare — it becomes home.

Some of my patients message me regularly through our patient portal. Updates, questions, musings. I don't always know what to say back. I don't walk on water. I'm trying my best. I make mistakes. I get tired. I sometimes wonder if I've done enough. Yet I don't downplay their gratitude, even if I don't feel worthy of it. Their belief in me is part of what keeps me going.

The Importance of Presence

Patients have told me I saved their life, that they wouldn't be here without me. The first time I heard that, I didn't know how to respond. What do you say when someone credits you with their existence? Thank you? I was just doing my job? Neither feels adequate. Because while I know medicine plays a role, I also know the truth: It's rarely just me. It's the patient's resilience, their family's support, the nurses and specialists who walk alongside us, the quiet hand of timing and chance. And yet, in their eyes, I was the difference between life and death.

Those words stay with me. They echo in the quieter moments of this work — the late nights charting, the mornings when exhaustion lingers, the days when the system feels heavier than the calling. They remind me why I chose this profession, why I keep choosing it.

Sometimes "saving a life" is catching a diagnosis before it's too late. Sometimes it's prescribing the right medication at the right dose. Other times, it's less obvious — it's sitting with someone in their despair long enough for them to decide to keep going. It's noticing the subtle pause before they answer, the heaviness in their tone, the way they almost — but not quite — admit they've lost hope. In those moments, listening can be as lifesaving as any procedure.

I don't think of myself as a savior. I think of myself as a witness. A guide. Someone who shows up when needed and who does their best to make the next step possible. But when a patient looks at me and says, "You saved my life," I realize that what feels routine to me may feel extraordinary to them.

It humbles me. It grounds me. It reminds me that medicine isn't about perfection — it's about presence. And sometimes, presence itself is what saves.

There's one patient I think of often. She had terminal cancer. She knew it. I knew it. We both understood that medicine had limits, that no treatment I could offer would reverse what her body was going through. And yet, she continued to come see me every month. Not because I could fix her, not because I had new answers, but because she wanted to talk.

One afternoon, she looked at me and said, "You've become part of my routine. You make me feel human." I've never forgotten those words. In a world where everything in her life revolved around her diagnosis — chemo schedules, scans, hospice conversations — our visits became something different. Not a treatment plan. Not a prognosis update. But a place where she wasn't just a patient with cancer — she was a person. That's something no test or treatment can measure.

Medicine often teaches us to focus on outcomes: survival rates, lab results, clinical milestones. But her presence reminded me that sometimes the most important outcome is simply being seen. Sometimes the most powerful intervention is presence itself — the steady reminder that even in decline, even in dying, a person still deserves dignity, connection, and to feel fully human.

I couldn't save her life. But maybe I gave her something else: a space where she could be more than her disease. And that, too, is medicine.

Not every story is easy. I've had patients lash out in anger, withdraw in silence, or spiral into despair. I've sat across from people who refused treatment, who cursed the system, who turned their frustration toward me because I was the one sitting in front of them. And yet, even in those difficult encounters, there's something to learn.

I've come to understand that anger is often fear in disguise. That silence can be a cry for help. That despair is not always a sign of weakness, but of someone carrying more than their share of life's weight. And I've learned that sometimes, the most healing thing I can offer is not a prescription, not a plan, not even an answer — but my presence. Simply sitting with someone, refusing to turn away, can be more powerful than any intervention.

Over time, my patients have become my teachers. They've taught me how to hold space for pain without rushing to fix it. How to celebrate small victories that might look insignificant on paper but mean everything in a life. How to grieve losses that aren't mine, yet feel personal because of the bond we share. How to set boundaries without building walls.

They've taught me patience. They've taught me humility. They've shown me that medicine isn't just about knowledge — it's about humanity. And in shaping the doctor I've become, they may have also shaped the man I'm still becoming.

We talk about the physician's role as one of authority, of expertise. Yet in truth, we're students as much as teachers. We're shaped by the people we serve. Their resilience, their vulnerability, their trust change us.

I may not have one defining patient story. What I have are a thousand small ones.

They aren't always dramatic. They don't all make headlines. But they've made me: A note slipped into my hand. A question asked in vulnerability. A tear shed in silence. A hug offered at the end of a visit. An update about a grandchild's graduation or a spouse's recovery.

Each moment has chipped away at the rigid edges of who I thought I had to be and has brought me closer to who I am.

It's not about a single story. It's about the mosaic of them all — the thousands of small, unglamorous, deeply human interactions that add up to a career, and more than that, a life.

The Choreography of Modern Medicine

I didn't choose primary care — it chose me. And now, looking back, I see that I haven't walked this journey alone. I've been walking it with a quiet army of teachers: my patients. The ones who stayed, the ones who left, the ones who visit even when they can barely walk.

If they ask me something about my life, about the system, about the process, I tell them. I talk about what it's like to be a doctor, a parent, a person navigating the chaos of modern medicine. I don't hide beneath the coat and the clicks. If anything, I try to open up — to show the human inside.

And yet, there are things about my life that I carry quietly, never saying them out loud — things I wish my patients knew.

I wish they knew how much I care. How much time I spend thinking about them — not just in the exam room, but on my drive home, in the middle of the night, while brushing my teeth. I wish they knew how often I carry their stories long after the visit is over. How invested I am in their outcomes even when the system makes it harder to show it.

I hear the questions in their voices:

Why haven't I heard about my lab results?

Why did my prescription take so long to get to the pharmacy?

Why couldn't I get in sooner when I was sick?

Why did the hospital say they never received the test you ordered?

The answers are rarely simple. Often they're layered in bureaucracy, delays, or breakdowns in communication. But the heart of the answers is this: Medicine has become a machine with too many moving parts. And many of those parts aren't designed to talk to each other.

When the gears jam or grind, the patient gets caught in the middle. But so do we. We feel the frustration too. We share the weight of the wait, the worry, the what-ifs. Behind every chart, every test, every prescription, is a physician who wishes their patient could see just how much they truly matter.

Medical assistants checking patients in, calling insurance companies, and trying to keep pace with a full schedule. Nurses managing messages, authorizations, and pre-visit planning. And me balancing it all while trying to remain fully present in the room, one patient at a time.

Behind every smooth encounter is a behind-the-scenes scramble. A front desk team coordinating appointments that change by the hour. Phones ringing, insurance forms faxing, portals crashing, prior authorizations stalled. Everyone working to make the impossible seem seamless.

A few years ago, a patient of mine needed a CT scan for unexplained weight loss. The order went in quickly, but the approval did not. Weeks passed. Every time I logged into the chart, the order still sat there — pending. My nurse spent hours on hold, my medical assistant called three different facilities when scheduling backlogs grew, and still we waited.

Finally, after relentless calls and paperwork, the scan was approved. By then, the patient had lost more weight, his anxiety growing with each day. When the results came back, the diagnosis was serious but treatable. We started care immediately.

What stays with me isn't the diagnosis — it's the delay. The way bureaucracy stood between a man and his health, and how easily he could have been lost in the shuffle. And the hard truth is this: It doesn't just happen once. It happens far too frequently. Different patient, different test, same barriers. Each time, the system stalls, and each time, it takes the persistence of a team to push through.

People imagine medicine as clean and efficient. The truth is, it runs on invisible acts of persistence. That CT scan didn't happen because of the system — it happened in spite of it.

Patients see me when the exam room door opens. What they don't see is the choreography behind it — the constant triage, the quiet negotiations, the dozens of invisible steps that make that one moment of connection possible.

Medicine looks simple from the outside: a conversation, a diagnosis, a prescription. But beneath the surface, it's a relay race of small, often thankless tasks that keep the system moving forward. It's the MA who calls three pharmacies until one finally has the medication in stock. It's the nurse who spends her lunch break fighting through hold music to secure an approval for an MRI. It's the front desk staff member who patiently reschedules the patient whose ride fell through for the third time this month.

These efforts don't show up in lab results or billing codes. They don't get documented in the chart. But they matter. Without them, the visit collapses; with them, care feels possible.

I often get the thanks — the handshake, the note, the appreciation. But the truth is, medicine isn't sustained by physicians alone. It's sustained by teams. By people whose names patients may never know, but whose work shapes every outcome.

When people picture medicine, they often imagine it as clean, precise, and efficient. Charts aligned. Labs delivered on time. Prescriptions sent without delay. A doctor walking in with answers. But the truth is, medicine is messy, improvisational. On the surface, everything looks orderly — like a cruise ship where meals arrive on time, the pool is clean, the music is playing. Yet beneath the surface, below deck, is an entirely different world. Crew members working double shifts, tightly coordinated operations, an entire ecosystem of labor you never see. They eat in different quarters, sleep in shared bunks, fix problems before they ever reach the top deck.

Outpatient medicine is no different. From the waiting room, it may look calm: Patients are checked in, rooms are ready, the doctor arrives with a smile. But below the surface is the unseen crew: Medical assistants juggling phone calls and intake forms, nurses pushing through endless prior authorizations, front desk staff troubleshooting schedules and insurance demands. The work is relentless, and much of it goes unnoticed.

My medical assistants arrive before I do and leave after I'm gone. They know my practice, sometimes better than I do. They can spot the patient who needs an extra-long visit before I've even opened the chart. They anticipate the lab I'll want to order before I order it. They notice the subtle change in a patient's weight or tone of voice and quietly flag it for me. They stay late to re-fax a prescription that got lost in transmission or call three pharmacies until they find one that actually has the medication in stock. When I'm running behind, they're the ones who keep patients calm, who explain what's happening, who make sure no one feels forgotten. They are the true heroes of my practice.

Like a ship, the clinic runs on invisible labor. The passengers see only the smooth ride. The reality is that every calm encounter in the exam room depends on a storm of effort behind the scenes — synchronized, exhausting, often thankless. And just like a ship's crew, when one person falls behind, the whole system feels it.

So when I think about the "system" of modern medicine, I try to remember it's not just a machine. It's a mosaic of people working tirelessly in the background. People who turn chaos into care. People who make it possible for me to walk into a room, sit down, and be fully present with my patient.

That's what patients rarely see: the army of hands that carry their care long before I ever walk in the room. Without that hidden work, the system would stall. With it, healing can happen.

My clinic uses one electronic health record. The hospital residency across the street uses another. They don't speak to each other. I might order a test, but unless I remember to fax the report or call directly, it won't be seen. That delay creates confusion, unnecessary repeat testing, and frustration for the patient, who simply wants answers.

And I don't blame them. I wish they knew I get frustrated too. I hate inefficiency. I hate when my hands are tied by bureaucracy. I hate calling an insurance company to fight for a prior authorization when I carry the truth that the test is necessary. I hate when I'm stuck documenting on a computer when I'd rather be talking face-to-face.

I wish my patients knew that the system is broken — but it's not their fault. It's not theirs to fix. It's ours to navigate.

We work inside a system that was never designed for ease, efficiency, or empathy. It's fragmented, outdated, and often more focused on metrics than meaning. And yet, we're expected to make it look effortless.

The burden of keeping things smooth falls on us. We're the ones holding the pieces together, patching the gaps, translating the mess into something that feels organized. Patients don't see the chaos because we're trained to shield them from it. But just because we make it look seamless doesn't mean it is.

I wish my patients knew that when their appointment runs behind, it's not because I don't value their time. It's because I'm giving the person before them the attention they deserve. And when it's their turn, they'll receive the same.

We're human. We make mistakes. But every single day, in a system that doesn't always make it easy, we show up and give our best.

And I'll be honest: There are days I go home feeling defeated. Not because of the patients, but because I carry the truth that I could have done more if I weren't fighting the clock, the paperwork, or the red tape. There are days I question whether I'm making a difference at all.

But then there are moments — quiet, human, healing moments — that cut through the noise. A patient who says, "Thank you for listening." A family that feels less alone after a hard conversation. A look of relief when someone realizes they've been heard, not rushed.

Those moments remind me why I started this work in the first place. They don't erase the chaos, but they make the fight worth it. These moments don't make headlines, but they make everything else bearable.

If I could tell my patients one thing, it would be this: I see you. I hear you. I care more than you know. I became a doctor to help people. And every day, even when it's hard — even when the system gets in the way — I'm trying to do that. So the next time something doesn't go as planned — when a call is delayed, or a message missed, or a follow-up falls through — know that behind the scenes, we're trying. We're below deck, keeping the ship afloat, even when the waters are rough.

Doing the Real Work

Medicine isn't perfect, yet neither is life. And like life, sometimes what matters most is that we're in it together.

I still remember the first time I had to deliver bad news. The fluorescent lights buzzed overhead, my white coat felt heavier than usual, and my mouth went dry as I sat across from a man whose life

I was about to change. The words "You have cancer" were on the tip of my tongue, but they felt impossible to say.

In that moment, I understood something textbooks never prepared me for: Medicine is not just science; it's the emotional aftermath. It's the silence that follows devastating news. It's the way your own stomach churns even as you steady your voice, because you know that your composure is the patient's last anchor.

I've carried that same tension in a thousand different ways. Walking into rooms where the fear is palpable. Watching families cling to hope when I know the prognosis is grim. Sitting at my desk long after the clinic is dark, wondering if I missed something, if I could have explained it better, if I could have done more.

That gnawing pit in the stomach? It never fully leaves. It's the fear of being wrong. Of failing. Of letting someone down. On the outside, I'm expected to be competent, confident, composed. On the inside, I've wrestled with the whisper: Am I good enough? Am I respected? Am I truly capable?

And then there are the difficult patients — the ones who test every ounce of patience and empathy I have left on a long day. Early in my career, I used to dread those encounters. But over time, I've realized that the patients who are the hardest to reach often become the most unforgettable. Sometimes frustration transforms into understanding, and understanding opens the door to connection.

I think of one patient who came in angry, distrustful, convinced no doctor cared. It would have been easy to match his defensiveness with my own. Instead, I listened. I learned about the years of being dismissed, the fear that no one was really hearing him. Slowly, that anger softened. Over months, we built a trust that neither of us expected.

That's the real work. Seeing not just the forest, but the trees — the leaves, the textures, the small, ordinary details of humanity. That's where medicine lives. Not only in the diagnosis, but in the presence we bring to another person's story.

I've come to understand that kindness can be taught, but genuineness takes time. It takes heart. It takes letting yourself be human enough to connect, even when vulnerability feels like a risk. Being a doctor means waking up never knowing exactly what the day will bring, and going home with questions that never fully quiet: Could I have done more? Said something differently? Did I miss the moment that mattered most?

That's the side of medicine we don't talk about enough. The self-doubt. The moral weight. The relentless pursuit of perfection — even though perfection is an illusion.

And yet, we show up every day. We adapt. We grow. We keep serving because it matters.

I remind myself often not to measure my worth by metrics, outcomes, or the finish line I can never quite reach. Instead, I look at the winding, imperfect path that brought me here — the setbacks, the doubts, the days I thought I couldn't keep going. Those moments are not proof of weakness. They're proof of resilience.

Because the truth is, many of the hardest challenges in medicine aren't rooted in pathology. They're rooted in fear — fear that shows up long before the diagnosis does. That's what we hold. That's what we walk with.

The Weight of the White Coat

Medicine has never asked me to be perfect; it has asked me to be present. To be human. And that's why I remind myself, again and again: My MD doesn't make me immune.

There's a dangerous myth that doctors are somehow immune — that the white coat shields us from the pain, fear, and vulnerability we spend our lives treating in others. As if the knowledge in our heads and the credentials on our walls are some kind of force field. Yet the truth is, we're human — fully, deeply, and sometimes painfully so.

I've lost count of how many times I've heard a variation of "You're a doctor. You must not get scared." Or "It must be easy for you to deal with this since you are a doctor." As if knowing makes feeling optional. It doesn't. If anything, knowledge can make it worse.

I don't float above illness; I walk through it, like everyone else. When my kids are sick, I feel helpless. I carry the knowledge — the signs, the symptoms, the risk factors — but it doesn't take away the ache in my chest when they cry, or the sleepless nights spent hovering outside their room, listening for the rise and fall of their breath. In those hours, I'm not a doctor. I'm a dad, scared and tired, wishing I could trade places with them.

When my wife isn't well, the roles blur in ways I never expected. Part of me wants to be the calm, informed spouse — the one who steadies the room and carries quiet certainty. But the truth is far less composed. My mind races through possibilities, drawing on knowledge I wish I didn't have. I can't turn it off. Every scenario, every complication, every outlier rushes forward, and suddenly I'm not the physician with perspective — I'm the husband who's scared.

The white coat doesn't help me there. If anything, it makes the weight heavier. It adds pressure to hold it all together, to be the anchor, to stay calm and unshaken — even when every part of me wants to crumble. The irony is that the knowledge I carry, the very thing that should empower me, often sharpens the fear instead. Because medicine doesn't make me immune. It only reminds me, over and over, just how fragile we all really are.

I carry the same responsibilities that so many of my patients do. I have aging parents and in-laws I worry about, wondering how to best support them as time does what it always does. I have bills that stack up, a mortgage that comes due every month, kids' activities that fill the calendar, and deadlines that don't care if I'm mentally exhausted. I have staff who rely on me to show up steady, patients who trust me to hold their stories, and a community that looks to me for guidance.

And yet, under all of that, I'm not just the doctor. I'm Ryan. A husband. A father. A son. A human being trying to carry it all, sometimes gracefully, sometimes not.

There's no immunity in this profession — only exposure. Deep, continuous exposure to suffering, complexity, and uncertainty. We see the frailty of the human body every day. We witness decline. We watch families shatter. And sometimes, we're the ones delivering the words that break them. That changes a person. It humbles you. It reshapes the way you walk through the world.

And when you find yourself on the other side of the exam table — whether as a patient, a parent, or a spouse — that perspective only deepens. My empathy is no longer just professional; it's personal. I don't just see my patients; I feel them. I know what it's like to wait for a call that doesn't come soon enough. To wonder if something important is being missed. To hope the labs come back normal and fear they won't. To feel like your concerns are either too big or not big enough.

That kind of knowing is heavy, but it's also what connects me most deeply to the people I care for. And so, I talk to my patients like people — because that's what they are. I tell them when I'm running behind, not out of guilt, but out of respect. I explain delays, not excuses. I share what I can about my own life when it feels appropriate. Sometimes it helps to remind them that I, too, am living this life, that I am not above it.

I wake up at 4 a.m. to work out. I go to my kids' soccer games. I show up at school concerts, at family dinners, and yes, at the pharmacy after hours when someone forgot to send a script. I try — impossibly sometimes — to balance everything. And I drop the ball sometimes. Not because I don't care, but because I'm human.

There's a unique kind of burnout that comes from having to pretend you're not allowed to feel. That you're supposed to be impenetrable. Yet the longer I've been in medicine, the more I've realized that vulnerability is not a weakness. It's a bridge.

When patients know I care — not just clinically, but personally — they open up. They let me in. And that's when the real healing begins.

Being vulnerable in medicine doesn't mean you're unstable. It means you're real. And realness is what this profession needs more of, not less.

I never want to forget what it feels like to be on the other side of the exam table. I never want the white coat to build walls. I want it to signal trust, yes, but also humanity, compassion, and presence. Because at the end of the day, I'm not Dr. Nadelson. I'm Ryan. A father. A husband. A son. A friend. A human being who happens to wear a white coat. And that white coat doesn't make me immune. It reminds me what's at stake.

In the Endings

Endings have a way of catching us off guard. In medicine, we often speak of beginnings — of first visits, new diagnoses, the hopeful start of a treatment plan. Yet I've found that the goodbyes carry their own quiet weight. And in many ways, they've taught me more than the introductions ever could.

Each time a patient walks through my door, I silently wonder: Will this be the last time I see them? It could be something as simple as a change in insurance. Or it could be something more final. Sometimes they quietly disappear from the schedule, and I never know why. Maybe they moved. Maybe they passed away. Maybe they found another physician. Maybe I wasn't the right fit for them.

Like anyone else, I want to be liked. I want to be respected. Needed. Trusted. I'd be lying if I said it doesn't sting when someone doesn't return and I don't know why. Was I too thorough? Not thorough enough? Too fast? Too slow? Too direct? Too quiet? Was it me?

In the early years, I obsessed over those thoughts. I took every goodbye personally. I believed that if I worked harder, studied more, tried to be everything to everyone, then no one would ever leave. But that's not how it works. Over time, I've come to realize this: You can't control how others see you. You can only control how you show up.

And many do see me. Many thank me. Some bring tears. Others share stories of how I helped change their lives in ways I never fully realized. A few have even found me years later, tracking me down through social media, sending a message just to say thank you. Some have come back to my office years after job changes, insurance changes, seeking out the doctor they remembered.

Those moments remind me that while not every connection lasts forever, the ones that do — even quietly, even from a distance — are the threads that hold me to this work. They are what make it worth it.

Over time, I've been gifted the chance to say goodbye more deliberately — to share that moment with patients who are moving away or transferring care. Those goodbyes are powerful. It's the highest form of validation when someone tells me they fought to come back. That they made the effort to reconnect. That they'd rather pay out-of-pocket than see someone else. In those moments, I carry the truth that I mattered — not because I was the smartest, not because I nailed the diagnosis, but because I was present, I listened, and I cared.

Of course, not every goodbye comes with such clarity. Sometimes you never get that final moment. And that, too, is part of the job: the ambiguity, the unknown, the quiet disappearances. You learn to accept that patients will leave your life as quietly as they entered it.

Still, the most difficult goodbyes haven't always been with patients. Some of them have been with colleagues, with family, with routines, with versions of myself.

Looking back, I've said goodbye to the young doctor who first walked into the outpatient clinic a decade ago — nervous, inexperienced, eager to prove himself. I remember that guy. He wanted to be liked more than he wanted to be trusted. He wanted to avoid mistakes more than he wanted to take risks. He wasn't yet sure of who he was, but he knew he wanted to matter.

Since then, I've said goodbye to that version of myself many times over.

I've grown into new versions — ones who are more confident, more grounded, more willing to admit what I don't know. I've let go of the need to be perfect. I have come to understand that humility and strength are not opposites. That listening is often more important than speaking. That patients don't always remember the details. But they remember how you made them feel.

I've said goodbye to the younger me who didn't know how to say no, who mistook burnout for dedication, who thought working longer hours always meant doing better work. I've said goodbye to the version of me who tied his self-worth too tightly to his productivity.

And I've welcomed new versions — more reflective, more balanced, more aware of what truly matters. I've become a husband. A father. A leader. A friend. Each role has brought new responsibilities, and each has required me to say goodbye to something else. Sometimes, it's a version of myself that I outgrew; other times, it's a season of life that has passed.

Each chapter in my life has taught me something, and with each goodbye, I have come to understand that endings are not failures — they're invitations. Invitations to reflect, to reset, to grow.

When you're young, you think goodbyes are sad. Yet as you grow, you realize they're necessary. They create space — for gratitude, for clarity, for transformation. They remind you that time is finite, that relationships are sacred. And that presence is the most precious gift you can offer another person.

So yes, I have come to understand a lot from saying goodbye.

I have come to understand to appreciate the patients who trusted me with their lives — even if only for a season.

I have come to understand to respect the colleagues who walked alongside me — and to let go when our paths diverged.

I have come to understand to embrace the discomfort of growth, to mourn the parts of myself I've outgrown — and to remain open to the person I am becoming.

And perhaps most importantly, I have come to understand that the most meaningful goodbyes are the ones that lead to better beginnings. For when you say goodbye with intention — with presence, with the act of being wholly there — and with gratitude, you leave the door open. Not just for others to return, but for yourself to move forward.

Beyond the Treatment

A man sat in my waiting room, his leg bouncing, his hand pressed to his chest. His heart wasn't racing from pain — it was panic. He'd spent the night Googling symptoms, scrolling through worst-case scenarios, convincing himself that something was fatally wrong. By the time I called his name, he wasn't just exhausted physically — he was drained emotionally.

I see this more and more. Patients don't come in empty anymore. They arrive with stories already written in their minds. Threads from online forums, posts from strangers, articles half-read at 2 a.m. By the time they reach me, it's not just their body that's tired — it's their spirit.

He wasn't the first. One patient once confessed, "I thought my low heart rate meant something serious. Like a rhythm issue. Maybe heart block." It wasn't. Just a normal variation. But fear has a way of swallowing logic whole.

Another whispered to me, eyes down, "I was worried you'd be disappointed... my blood pressure crept up. I tried so hard." The numbers were fine. What startled me wasn't the reading — it was the shame. The belief that they had somehow failed me. I've never scolded a patient for a number. In fact, I've never scolded a patient at all. Medicine, to me, has never been about blame — it's about partnership. We're in this together.

And I understand their fear more than they know. Because I've lived it too.

I remember one night standing in the doorway of my daughter's room, listening for the rise and fall of her breath. She had spiked a fever earlier that day, and though every part of me knew the guidelines, knew the probabilities, knew the odds were in her favor, my chest still tightened with worry. I stood there in the dark, holding my own breath, waiting for the reassurance of hers. In that moment, I wasn't a physician. I was a father — afraid of the same unknowns that haunt my patients.

I've refreshed lab portals late at night, staring at results I could recite in my sleep, yet still feeling that knot in my stomach. I've waited on phone calls I knew might not come until morning. I've let my mind race through every possibility, from the common to the catastrophic. Even as a doctor, when it's me or someone I love, knowledge doesn't shield me — it sharpens the edge of uncertainty.

I once saw a woman panic over a mild bump in her liver enzymes. "Was it the glass of wine I had the night before?" she asked. "The Tylenol for my headache? Could it be cancer?" She had cycled through every explanation. The reality? A harmless, temporary blip. What she needed wasn't a prescription. She needed context. She needed compassion. In 60 seconds, I could offer her something Google never would: reassurance.

That's why, when I walk into a room, I try to start with presence. I ask about their family, their vacation, their week. I smile. I listen. I want them to know they're not a lab result. They're not a number on a page. And they're not in trouble.

Because I've come to believe we don't just treat disease. We treat doubt. We treat fear. We treat the space between what could be and what is.

There are days I wish I could write a prescription for peace of mind as easily as I can for blood pressure. But it doesn't work that way. Peace isn't ordered; it's built. It's built on trust, communication, and the simple act of being present.

The truth is, in modern medicine, illness isn't always the hardest part. It's the waiting. The what if. The silence between visits. The fear that maybe something's being missed. And sometimes, the most powerful medicine we can offer isn't what we prescribe — it's what we say.

In medicine, we're taught to focus on facts — labs, imaging, diagnoses, treatment plans. Yet the longer I practice, the more I realize that the true art of healing lies somewhere else. It lies in connection, history, meaning, and moments. And more than anything, it lies in the relationships we build over time.

I've met patients who remember when Coca-Cola cost five cents and when movie tickets were a quarter. They remember a time before the internet, before television, before modern medicine looked anything like it does today. I've had the privilege of caring for patients who span generations — from those turning 18 to those nearing 100. It's a gift that not many professions offer: a front-row seat to nearly a century of lived experience.

Times have changed. Prices have changed. Perspectives have changed. Yet the human need for connection? That hasn't changed at all.

Pieces of Themselves

What's amazed me most over the years is not what I've been able to give my patients, but what they've chosen to give me.

Patients bring more than their stories — they bring keepsakes, pieces of themselves, physical reminders of lives well lived. Over the years, I've quietly built a small collection of these sentimental treasures. A basket of mementos now sits in the corner of my office — not as decoration, but as a tribute to the relationships I've built and the people who have entrusted me with fragments of their past.

At first, I didn't know what to do with them. A gift offered in passing. A token of gratitude. A small object pressed into my hand as if to say: I trust you enough to share this part of me. I could have tucked them away in drawers, but that felt wrong. To hide them would be to diminish their meaning. And so they sit where I can see them, not for show, but as a reminder of what medicine really is.

These small, powerful gestures speak volumes. They're unexpected. They're humbling. And they remind me, again and again, that what we do in medicine goes far beyond prescriptions and protocols. We're not just treating illness — we're sharing in people's lives.

I think about how rare that kind of trust is. Most people don't invite their accountant into their living room. They don't tell their lawyer about their childhood fears. They don't bring their financial adviser a jar of homemade jam. But doctors live in that in-between space: professional, yet personal; clinical, yet deeply human. We're part of people's stories in a way that defies easy explanation.

I don't pretend that every patient relationship is easy. Some are complicated, some never find their rhythm, but the ones that do — the ones that blossom into trust, connection, and gratitude — are the heart of this work. The gifts remind me that even in a healthcare system obsessed with efficiency, metrics, and productivity, the soul of medicine is still personal.

I used to feel conflicted about accepting these gifts. Was it appropriate? Was it professional? But over time, I realized that refusing them wasn't humility — it was dismissal. These weren't "things"; they were stories. To reject them would be to say your gesture doesn't matter. And it does matter — sometimes more than the lab I ordered or the prescription I refilled.

One patient told me, "You listened to me when no one else did." He left me with a small keepsake from his desk, nothing of material value, but heavy with meaning. That gift wasn't about me; it was about the relief of finally being heard.

I think of these objects as touchstones. On the hard days — when the charting piles up, when the insurance battles drag on, when the system feels like it's grinding me down — I turn toward the basket in the corner of my office. It grounds me. Each item in it holds a story, a relationship, a reminder that what I do matters beyond lab values and prescriptions.

When I feel worn thin by the endless pace of modern medicine, that basket reminds me of the humanity that still threads through this work. It reminds me that medicine is not sustained by efficiency or metrics, but by connection. That people don't remember how many clicks I logged or how fast I closed a chart — they remember whether I was present, whether I listened, whether I cared.

And in those moments of exhaustion, it gives me perspective. It helps me remember that I'm not defined by the battles I lose against the system, but by the moments of trust I earn within it. That quiet collection of mementos is more than decoration; it's a compass, pointing me back to why I chose this life in the first place.

Because medicine is not only about curing. It's about witnessing. It's about standing alongside people in their most vulnerable moments and saying, I see you. I care. You matter.

These gifts don't live on a shelf because they're beautiful. They live there because they anchor me. They remind me that even when I feel like I'm failing the system, I'm not failing the people who matter most. They remind me that presence can heal, even when the science runs out.

In the end, I don't think patients bring gifts because they believe I need more things. They bring them because they want me to know that our time together mattered. That I mattered. And in giving them, they remind me of the most important truth of all:

The best medicine isn't always written on a pad. Sometimes, it's found in a simple act of gratitude. Sometimes, it's carried in a basket in the corner of the room.

And when patients see me as more than their doctor — when they see me as an equal, a confidant, an extended part of their family

— they let down their guard. They exhale. They feel safe. That's when the real stories surface, the fears they've been carrying, the questions they were too nervous to ask anywhere else.

Counting My Blessings

Some of my most medically complex patients — the ones juggling multiple specialists, medications, and worries that never quite leave — have told me they feel more at ease in my exam room than anywhere else. Hearing that is one of the greatest honors I could ever receive.

Because in the end, it's not just about solving the medical puzzle. It's about creating a space where someone feels human again, even in the midst of their illness.

Being uncomfortable? That's a terrible feeling. It's isolating. It's overwhelming. And it has no place in the healing process. My goal is always to create a space where people feel seen, heard, and respected — no matter their background, no matter their condition.

Medicine is not a hierarchy. It's not about power. It's not about barking orders or rushing through charts. It's about sitting down, looking someone in the eye, and saying: "I see you. I'm here for you. Let's figure this out together."

Many of my patients in their 80s and 90s have seen things I could hardly imagine. Some grew up in the shadow of the Great Depression, remembering nights when dinner was bread, beans, and little else. Some fought in World War II or waited at home for telegrams that could change everything. I've heard stories of men who stormed beaches, women who worked in factories, and families who scraped together ration coupons just to get sugar for a holiday cake.

Others lived through segregation, recalling a time when entire communities were divided by lines they had no choice but to follow. A few tell me about polio outbreaks, about classmates who vanished from school and never returned.

Some carry scars far deeper than illness. I've cared for Holocaust survivors who described being children when the world turned on them — when neighbors disappeared, when families were separated, when survival meant enduring hunger, hiding in silence, or being forced onto trains bound for unthinkable places. They sit across from me decades later, still gentle, still dignified, and I am humbled by the weight of what they endured.

They remember first televisions, black-and-white sets glowing in darkened living rooms. They remember when doctors made house calls, when milk was delivered to the doorstep, when Sunday dinners stretched across three generations at the table. And when they sit across from me — frail bodies, sharp memories — I realize I'm not just listening to patients. I'm listening to living history.

We talk a lot about the burdens of medicine: burnout, bureaucracy, documentation. And those are real. They wear on us, they sap our energy, and some days they make us wonder why we ever chose this path.

Yet the blessings? They're just as real, and far too often overlooked. The blessing of being trusted with someone's fears. Of being invited into the most private corners of a person's life. The blessing of sitting with an 85-year-old who tells me about his time in World War II, and then turning to a 20-year-old navigating anxiety in a world the veteran could never have imagined. The blessing of witnessing the arc of life, from first checkups to final breaths, and knowing that in those moments, presence matters more than perfection.

The system will always make this work hard. But the relationships — the stories, the keepsakes, the simple words of "thank you for listening" — are what keep me grounded. They're what transform a profession into a calling.

The blessings are in the tiny moments. The stories passed down. The gifts given without expectation. The hugs after hard diagnoses. The relief in someone's eyes when they know they've been heard.

When someone gives me something they've held onto for decades — a keepsake, a note, a memory — it's not about the object. It's about the trust. The connection. The sentiment. For if it's sentimental to them, it's sentimental to me.

And that's the part of medicine they don't teach you in training. The part that doesn't show up in your board scores or your EMR documentation. The part that's rooted not in science. But in humanity. I'll never take that for granted.

Putting Up the Bumpers

When you're a kid, they put up the bumpers at the bowling alley — not to guarantee a strike every time, but to keep the ball from falling off course completely. The bumpers don't steer the ball or control the outcome — they just keep it in play.

The bumpers are quiet, steady. They're always there — not to interfere, but to guide.

That's how I think of my childhood.

My mom and dad were always there for me — my biggest supporters. They showed up at games, at school events, at graduations. They never missed the moments that mattered. But just as important as their presence was the way they gave me space. They were close enough that I knew I was safe, but not so close that I felt smothered. They let me breathe. They let me grow. They let me stumble and scrape my knees without rushing in to carry me off the lane.

Looking back, I realize how much of who I became was shaped not by dramatic interventions but by quiet guardrails. Their love wasn't about micromanaging me into success. It was about creating an environment where I could fail safely, recalibrate, and try again. That steady, quiet kind of love was the foundation that carried me forward.

I think of my dad's calm encouragement — rarely flashy, never overbearing. He wasn't one to push his voice above others, but his steady presence spoke volumes. When I doubted myself, he'd say just enough to remind me that I had what it took. He didn't force the ball down the lane; he just kept me from falling into the gutter.

I think of my mom's constant belief in me — her unwavering faith that I could handle whatever came my way. She never stood over my shoulder demanding perfection. She just reminded me, again and again, that I was capable. Her support wasn't loud, but it was fierce. When I think about the bumpers in bowling, I picture her there — always close, always protective, yet never robbing me of the chance to take the shot myself.

That balance — the combination of presence and space — is what allowed me to grow into my own life. And it's a balance I carry with me now, both as a parent and as a physician.

As a father, I think about how tempting it can be to hover. To rush in and fix every frustration my kids face. But then I remember how much I learned from the small stumbles; how the lessons I still carry weren't born of being shielded from struggle, but from being supported through it. My parents trusted me to find my own way within safe boundaries. That trust gave me confidence. I want my kids to feel that same combination of security and freedom. I want to be their bumpers.

As a physician, I've come to realize that the best kind of guidance works the same way. Patients don't need me to live their lives for them. They don't need me to micromanage every decision. They need me to walk alongside them, to set the boundaries of safety, and to support them when they start to veer off track. They need reassurance that they're not alone, but also the space to make their own choices.

When I think about how my parents raised me, I see echoes in my exam room. My role isn't to control the outcome; it's to keep the ball in play; to offer steady, quiet support; to let people breathe, grow, and own their decisions while knowing they're not abandoned.

The world often tells us that love means control, that success means managing every detail, that failure means we've done something wrong. But my parents taught me the opposite. They taught me that love is presence without suffocation; that success is learning from the wobble as much as from the strike; that failure isn't the end of the game — it's just another roll of the ball.

Medicine often tempts us toward control. We want to solve everything, fix everything, tie every loose end. But real healing doesn't come from domination; it comes from partnership. It comes from being the bumpers: quiet, steady, always there.

And the same is true in parenting. My kids will have their own paths. They'll drift, they'll struggle, they'll surprise me in ways I can't predict. My job isn't to script their every move. My job is to keep them in play.

When I sit with patients, when I sit with my children, I find myself drawing on the same lesson my parents gave me: Be close enough to catch them, but far enough to let them roll. Love them fiercely, but quietly. Guide without controlling. Support without suffocating.

That's the kind of parenting that shaped me. That's the kind of medicine I want to practice. And that's the kind of life I want to live: walking the lane with my family, with my patients, with anyone who trusts me to stand beside them.

Because in the end, the goal isn't a perfect strike every time. The goal is to stay in play. And for that, the bumpers matter more than we realize.

Looking back, I realize how much of who I became was shaped not by big corrections, but by those subtle guardrails. Their presence gave me space to make mistakes, to find my own momentum, while still knowing I wouldn't be lost.

They didn't micromanage my move or chart a rigid course I had to follow. They didn't hover over my homework, dictate my future, or demand perfection. Instead, they provided structure without suffocation, encouragement without expectation, love without condition.

They were always there, gently nudging me back when I veered too far off course. If I made a mistake, I wasn't scolded — I was taught. If I fell short, I wasn't punished — I was given the space to learn and try again. And when I succeeded, it wasn't met with "Finally" — it was met with pride, with warmth, with presence.

I wasn't an Ivy League student. I didn't graduate at the top of my class. I wasn't some academic prodigy with a perfect test score and a flawless résumé. I struggled at times. I doubted myself. I stumbled through school trying to find my rhythm. Yet I had a clear goal: I wanted to become a doctor.

They never made me believe that one version of success was the only version worth pursuing. They didn't look down on me for going to a Caribbean medical school. If anything, they admired my persistence, my grit, my unwillingness to give up because the path was different.

That dream never changed. And no matter how imperfect the path became, my parents never let me forget that the goal was valid, possible. They never made me feel like my dreams had to come with credentials. That's something I carry with me every day.

For here's the truth: I've never viewed myself as the best at anything. I wasn't the fastest runner, the smartest kid in the room, or the most popular guy at school. I was ordinary, average. Yet in a way, that made me more grounded. I learned early on that being good enough — being consistent, being kind, being steady — could carry you as far as chasing greatness.

I wasn't babied. When I messed up, I heard about it. If I said something I shouldn't have, I was corrected. If I slacked off or did poorly in school, my parents noticed. Yet they didn't make me feel like less of a person. I was never grounded for weeks or made to feel ashamed. Discipline in our house was never about power. It was about growth.

That's the lesson that stuck. You don't need fear to teach responsibility. You don't need shame to create accountability. You need honesty, love, and consistency.

Now, as a parent, I see those same principles come through in the way I raise my own kids.

Farah and I aren't authoritarian. We know they're going to make mistakes. We know they're going to push back, test limits. And sometimes say or do the wrong thing. That's what kids do. That's how they grow.

We have rules, sure. Expectations. Boundaries. Yet we also have understanding. We have room. We have patience. For we know that failure is part of learning. That struggle is part of growth. That discipline doesn't need to break you to be effective.

When our kids get a bad grade, we don't yell. We talk. We ask what happened. We help them figure out what they didn't understand. When they act out or say something unkind, we don't shame them. We hold them accountable and teach them how to do better. When they fall short, we don't define them by the mistake. We define them by how they respond.

We are not raising perfect kids. We're raising real ones. Kids who stumble, who test limits, who get it wrong and then try again. Kids who need room to fall short so they can discover how to stand tall.

Perfection was never the goal. Presence was. Consistency was. Love was. And if my children grow up knowing they are seen, supported, and trusted — even in their messiness, even in their imperfection — then I'll know I've done my job.

We want them to know that it's okay to stumble. It's okay to feel lost. It's okay to not always get it right the first time. We want them to roll freely — without fear.

That's the power of the bumpers. They don't take away the effort. They don't change the game. They create a safe environment for you to grow, to try, to fall and try again. They keep you from falling so far off the lane that you stop believing in yourself.

That's what my parents gave me, and that's what I want to give my kids.

It's funny: When you're a kid, you don't think much about the bumpers. You don't realize the safety they provide or the intention behind them. You're just glad they're there. Yet as an adult, I see them so clearly now — the way my parents protected me from the harshness of perfectionism, the way they gave me permission to be human, to explore, to fail, to find my own voice. And that's what I hope my kids will remember, too.

Not the rules we set — but the grace behind them.

Not the lectures — but the conversations.

Not the pressure — but the presence.

What I want most is for my kids to look back and feel that we believed in them — not only when they succeeded, but especially when they struggled. Because that's when belief matters most. It's easy to cheer from the sidelines when the score is high, when the grades are perfect, when the outcome looks polished. But the real test of love is standing steady when the ball drifts, when the lane feels uneven, when the strike never comes.

That's what the bumpers are for. That's what parenting, at its best, is.

Rapport, Respect, and Relationships

Rapport is defined as a close and harmonious relationship in which people understand each other's feelings and communicate with mutual respect. In medicine, it's the intangible connection that makes a patient feel seen, heard, and cared for — not just treated. Rapport is about relationship building. About connection.

I try to begin building that connection within the first 30 seconds of meeting someone. A simple smile, steady eye contact, a handshake — even a shared laugh — can change the entire tone of the visit. Those small gestures set the stage for trust. They send a quiet but unmistakable message: I'm here. I see you. I care.

Over the years, I've learned that patients don't always remember every detail of what I explained or prescribed, but they always remember how they felt in the room with me. Did they feel rushed? Or did they feel respected? Did they feel like a case? Or did they feel like a person? Rapport is what makes the difference.

First impressions matter — and they're not one-way. I pay attention to how the patient responds to the handshake, to the greeting, to the small talk. If something doesn't land — if the interaction feels off — I pivot. I take a different route. I shift the tone, the language, the approach. Reading the room isn't an optional skill in medicine; it's part of the job.

And that's where rapport starts: not with credentials, but with presence.

When people think about what makes a "good doctor," they often point to the usual markers: where you went to medical school, what institution you're affiliated with, how many letters follow your name. And while those things may carry weight on paper, they mean little if you can't connect in the exam room. Patients don't measure competence by diplomas on the wall; they measure it by how you make them feel — whether you listen, whether you respect them, whether they can finally exhale when they're with you.

The truth is, patients rarely care about the pedigree. They don't come in asking about rankings or résumés. What they do care about — what builds trust, what keeps them coming back — is rapport, that subtle, fragile, powerful bond that says "You're safe here, you matter here, you're more than a chart or a lab result."

I've found the most underrated but powerful way to build that rapport is simple: Be yourself.

You don't need to act. You don't need to put on a hyper-professional mask that hides who you are as a person. In fact, I'd argue you shouldn't. Patients can spot a performance from a mile away. They know when you're guarded, distracted, or checked out. Just like they know when you're fully present, honest, and real.

Being yourself doesn't mean being unfiltered or harsh. It means being emotionally available and authentic. It means showing you care — even when that care includes being direct.

Sometimes honesty requires us to deliver uncomfortable truths. Not to be mean or critical, but to advocate for what the patient truly needs. And if you've built the kind of rapport where communication flows with mutual respect, those messages land; they make an impact, changes get made, and health improves.

Other times? Not so much. And that's where the part of medicine with no ICD code takes over. It's not about knowledge — it's about emotional intelligence, adaptability, and knowing how to read the room. You learn when to soften your tone, when to lean in with confidence, when to let silence do the work. That kind of skill doesn't show up on a résumé, but it often defines the quality of your care more than anything else.

Building rapport requires finesse. Some patients are naturally easy to talk to; others take more time. Time and again, I've walked into exam rooms and made a split-second decision on how to approach the conversation.

Does this patient have a sense of humor? Are they more serious? Are they married, widowed, single? Are they young, or are they elderly? Each of these details shifts how I communicate — and I have only seconds to adapt.

It's something I do daily, across all kinds of visits. And over the years, through sheer repetition, I've learned how to read the room — how to sense what's appropriate to say and what's better left unsaid. It's not easy, and it doesn't happen overnight.

If you're a new physician — or still figuring it out — don't be hard on yourself. This isn't something taught in textbooks. It's a skill that can only be acquired with time, patience, and experience. That's the invisible art of human communication. And when you learn to navigate it, medicine becomes something more than a job. It becomes a relationship.

Today, I can walk into a room and connect with patients from all walks of life: young and old, affluent and underserved, English-speaking and not — even through a translator. I've talked with colleagues, teenagers, grandparents, and each interaction requires something different. What matters most isn't the script you walk in with, but the willingness to adapt, to meet someone where they are, to speak in a way that makes them feel seen.

That's when the walls come down. That's when medicine moves beyond charts and protocols into something deeply human.

I often say that talking to a patient should feel no different than talking to a loved one. If you feel strongly about something, say it. If you have clear guidance, offer it. Patients want that. They trust you. They rely on your judgment. And when they believe that you truly care, they're far more likely to listen.

After a decade in primary care, I've noticed something: A lot of doctors feel like they can't break character. That being "too human" in the room is somehow unprofessional. That showing emotion might be interpreted as a sign of weakness.

But weakness to who? Because I can tell you that patients don't see it that way. If anything, it's the opposite. When you show emotion, when you speak with passion, when you let them see that you care, it doesn't diminish your authority. It deepens your connection. It shows strength, not weakness.

The truth is that people don't want perfect doctors. They want present ones. They don't remember the flawless delivery of a diagnosis; they remember whether you sat with them in the silence that followed. They don't measure you by whether your voice cracked; they measure you by whether you were willing to stay when theirs did.

That's not a loss of professionalism. That's the heart of medicine. Medicine is human. We sit face-to-face with people navigating incredible highs and devastating lows, and sometimes, we find ourselves right there in the middle of it. That's okay.

The barrier we think we have to keep up — that wall of stoicism and detachment — doesn't always need to stay standing. You can be human. You can show empathy. In fact, your patients want it. They deserve it. To them, you're not just a prescriber or a problem-solver. You're their mentor. Their medical guide. Their liaison through some of the hardest, and often most meaningful, moments of their lives.

And at the core of that connection? Trust. Respect. And the smallest of choices we make along the way — sometimes as simple as the name we choose to be called.

That's why rapport isn't "nice to have." It's an outpatient clinical tool. A force multiplier. It makes your advice actionable. Your presence — meaningful. Your care — memorable.

So yes, it might mean coming out of your shell a bit. That's not a flaw in your practice — it's the heart of it. Because before we treat the patient, we have to meet the person.

A Question of Comfort

In medicine, one surprisingly heated debate doesn't get much airtime: Should patients call their doctors by their first name?

It pops up often on medical forums. I've seen long threads dissect whether it's disrespectful, whether it undermines authority, or whether it simply reflects a cultural shift in how we view physicians. Some doctors insist on "Doctor" as a matter of principle — status, respect, professionalism.

Me? I appreciate being called Dr. Nadelson. It reflects the role I play and the responsibility I carry. Yet if someone calls me "Ryan," I'm not the least bit perturbed. My parents named me Ryan. To my friends, my colleagues, and my family, I'll always be Ryan. I happened to earn a medical degree. In the exam room, yes, I'm Dr. Nadelson. The title matters. It marks the professional trust I hold. But outside of that? I'm me.

I worked hard for the degree, and I'm proud of it. Yet when a patient uses my first name, I don't see it as disrespect. I often take it as a sign of comfort — maybe even trust. If that small gesture helps someone feel more at ease, opens them up, or makes the room feel more human, then I welcome it. Because in the end, the title may signal knowledge, but the name signals connection. And sometimes, connection is the most powerful medicine we can offer.

Some physicians believe we should call patients "Mr." or "Ms." followed by their last name. I understand the intent: it's polite and professional. Yet to me, it can feel distant. Cold. Like we're keeping a barrier in place. My patients aren't names on a chart. They're part of my work family. I see them regularly. So if they call me Ryan, I don't correct them. I don't need a title to feel secure in my role. I'm here to listen, to guide, to heal — not to be placed on a pedestal.

This is personal for many doctors. I've seen it spark strong reactions. And I respect that. If "Doctor" matters to you, say so. Set that boundary. It's valid. For me, though, I've found that "Ryan" opens more doors than it closes. Some patients say "Mr. Ryan." Others call me "Mr. Nadelson." I don't take offense. I'm grateful they remember my name at all. That alone tells me we've connected, that something about our time together mattered enough to stick.

To be clear, I'm not dismissing anyone who prefers "Doctor." The title carries meaning, history, and weight. But I don't believe anything less than that automatically signals disrespect or weakens the physician–patient bond. For me, it's not the title that builds trust; it's the relationship that grows in the space between us — the listening, the presence, the care.

In formal settings — team rounds, hospital residency meetings, academic discussions — titles have their place. They add structure and clarity. In the exam room, where relationships build over years, familiarity can create trust in ways formality never could.

In many communities, first names aren't a slight. They're a sign of warmth. And let's be honest — we call patients by their first names all the time. Maybe they're reflecting that back. Are some patients trying to level the playing field? Maybe. Asserting a bit of control in a vulnerable moment? Possibly. Saying, "Let's be human together?" Absolutely.

And if that's what comes from using my first name, I'll take it every time. And that's why I don't take it personally. It means the white coat didn't build a wall. It means the power dynamic didn't block connection. It means I'm doing something right.

Respect matters. And yes, the title "Doctor" carries weight. But I've come to believe respect isn't found in what people call you — it's in how they treat you. It's in whether they trust you, whether they feel safe with you, whether they believe you'll show up for them when it matters most. It's whether they listen when you speak.

I didn't become a doctor to be addressed differently. I became one to make a difference. So yes, I appreciate being called Dr. Nadelson. It honors the work, the training, and the trust. Yet if someone calls me Ryan, I won't correct them. I'll meet them where they are. Because comfort, openness, and trust matter more to me than formality ever could.

As much as we focus on the exam room, we can't ignore the system that surrounds it and the ways it strains those within it. But behind every title is a person. A human being navigating the same struggles, the same hopes, the same desire to connect.

And maybe that's the point. The title acknowledges the role. The name acknowledges the person. Both matter. But it's the humanity that endures.

Doctors aren't immune to burnout or doubt, and we need to stop pretending they are. Support means more than applause; it means change. And when patients remember that — when they see the human beneath the coat and the clicks — that's when healing truly begins.

The Currency of Medicine

Medicine is built on relationships. Yes, it's about science and systems and protocols, but at its core, it's about people learning from and leaning on each other. And that learning? It often follows a simple, timeless principle: tit for tat.

In game theory, tit for tat means reciprocity — matching what's given, responding in kind. In medicine, I've found it works the same way. When I offer openness, patients respond with honesty. When I bring respect, they return it. When I show vulnerability, they often meet me with their own. Over time, those small exchanges build something far bigger than information — they build trust.

And trust is the currency of medicine. Without it, even the best science falls flat. With it, even the hardest truths can be heard.

When I show up engaged, curious, and ready to learn, my attendings are more likely to teach. When I ask thoughtful questions, take ownership of my patients, and demonstrate respect for the process, I tend to receive more guidance in return. That exchange isn't always verbalized. It's subtle, but powerful. It builds trust and fuels growth.

And it doesn't stop with training. Reciprocal learning shows up in the quiet moments: asking a peer how they handle a difficult conversation or how they talk someone through a devastating diagnosis. It's offering advice on navigating a complicated insurance appeal and knowing that when your turn comes, someone will step up for you too.

In practice, reciprocity is everywhere. It lives in the culture of medicine at its best. It's in colleagues trading call coverage — not because they have to, but because they care. It's in the nurse who goes the extra mile for your patient, and in the way you return the favor when her day is stretched thin. It's in the resident who stays late to help with an admission, trusting that someday, someone else will stay late for them.

This give-and-take, this rhythm of leaning on each other, is the engine that keeps the profession moving forward. It's not written in any protocol, but it's what sustains us when the system feels like it won't.

Residency is often the first place we see it clearly. We cover for each other. We share resources. We stay late to help with admissions or work through a challenging differential. Not because it's required, but because we know it'll come back around. We're not keeping score. We're building a team.

And still, even more than a team, we're building something bigger: a profession rooted in mutual respect. Those late nights, those small sacrifices, those moments of stepping in when someone else is stretched too thin — they're not just acts of kindness. They're the glue that holds the culture of medicine together.

That spirit doesn't disappear after training — it just takes new forms. In outpatient practice, reciprocity looks different, but it's no less important. It's the colleague who covers your panel when you're out with the flu and you returning the favor months later. It's a medical assistant stepping in to calm an anxious patient, knowing you'll support her when she's overwhelmed by phone calls and refills. It's a nurse flagging a detail you almost missed and you making sure to recognize her contribution in front of the team.

Even the patients teach me reciprocity. They remind me that when I listen closely, they listen back. When I take the time to explain, they trust the plan. When I show compassion, they return it in ways I never expect: through kindness, gratitude, even the small keepsakes they leave behind in my office.

Reciprocal learning and reciprocal care are what make this profession sustainable. Without them, medicine feels transactional. With them, it becomes what it was always meant to be: a shared human endeavor. You give, I take. I take, you give. It's not transactional. It's collaborative. It's the glue that holds our teams, our systems, and our patient care together.

No one practices medicine in isolation. Whether in a hospital residency or in the outpatient setting, we rely on one another across specialties, across disciplines, across roles. Primary care physicians are often the gatekeepers. We open the door, initiate the referral, start the workup. But that's only the beginning. What follows is a chain of mutual responsibility, accountability, and trust. The cardiologist depends on the history I've gathered. The physical therapist builds on the goals we've set. The pharmacist ensures the plan is safe and sustainable. Each step is tied to the one before and the one after, bound by reciprocity.

And when it works, it's seamless. The patient may not even see the handoffs, the back-and-forth phone calls, the quiet teamwork happening behind the scenes. But that's the point. Reciprocity is most powerful when it's invisible — when it feels less like a transaction and more like a shared commitment to someone else's well-being.

When I refer a patient to a specialist, I trust they'll receive thoughtful, expert care. In return, I hope that specialist will communicate clearly, send the patient back, and keep me in the loop. That give-and-take isn't about ego. It's about efficiency, respect, and what's best for the patient. When that loop works the way it should, it feels seamless. It strengthens care. It strengthens relationships.

And it's not just about the clinical handoff; it's cultural. Reciprocity is the backbone of professionalism. It builds trust among physicians, nurtures respect between primary care and specialists, and creates bridges between attendings and trainees, administrators, and clinicians. Everyone has a role. Everyone brings value. And when that value is recognized and reciprocated, the whole system works better.

Of course, we don't always say it out loud. There's no formal agreement. There is an understanding: If I cover your patient today, you'll have my back tomorrow. If I support your judgment in a difficult case, you'll do the same for me. If I go the extra mile to coordinate care, I trust that effort won't go unnoticed.

This dynamic shows up with patients, too. The more I respect them, listen without judgment, and offer honest guidance, the more they lean in. They trust me. They open up. They follow through. They come back. It's not about authority or titles; it's about partnership.

That reciprocity is subtle, but it's powerful. When I give my full attention, they give me their truth. When I show them I care, they show me their effort. That cycle — built on presence, not prescription — creates the kind of healing no lab test can measure.

Reciprocal learning is not confined to academic conferences or feedback sessions. It lives in the small moments. The five-minute curbside consult in the hallway. The brief chat after outpatient clinic about how to handle burnout. The resident who takes the time to explain something to a medical student because someone once did the same for them.

It's mentorship in motion. It's support without strings attached. It's the unspoken agreement that we're in this together — and when I help you, I'm not losing anything; I'm building something.

In a system that often feels fragmented, impersonal, and rushed, this kind of reciprocity grounds us. It reminds us why we chose this field in the first place. It reminds us that at the end of the day, we're all here for the same reason: to care for our patients and each other.

So yes, medicine is science. Yet it's also a social contract. A culture. A practice of mutual respect.

And when we engage in reciprocal learning — when we teach, support, and show up for each other — we don't just become better doctors, we become better people. We become colleagues who listen more deeply, mentors who lift instead of judge, teammates who step in without being asked. We build a profession not on hierarchy alone, but on humility, trust, and shared humanity.

Because in the end, what sustains us isn't the individual victories. It's the network of hands that steady us when we stumble, and the moments when we do the same for someone else.

The Rhythm of the Profession

You know that feeling when you've got the number: the patient count, the packed schedule, the full inbox? It's not panic — it's something else. Almost excitement. You're gearing up for something demanding. Something important.

It's not a high, but it's definitely a shift. Surreal, maybe. Like your body starts preparing before your brain does. There's a tightening in your chest, a mental bracing. You're not even at the office yet, but your body knows: it's game time.

I've felt that rhythm so many mornings. The drive in, hyped up on my coffee, rehearsing the day before it begins. Who needs a medication refill? Who's following up on a scare from the ER? Who's waiting for results that could alter the course of their life? The list is long, and before the first patient even walks through the door, you're already in motion.

It's a strange kind of readiness — part adrenaline, part muscle memory, part quiet determination. Your mind sharpens, scanning through possibilities before they even arrive. You've got the faces memorized, the stories recalled, the loose ends waiting to be tied. By the time you sit at your desk, you're already two steps into the day.

There's no easing in, no gentle warm-up. The rhythm starts immediately. A lab result flashes on the screen, a refill request pops up, a voicemail is waiting to be returned. Even before the first knock on the door, you're bracing for the inevitable shift from preparation to presence. That moment when a patient walks in and the lists, the inbox, the paperwork all fall away because right then, it's just you and them.

It's not glamorous, and it's not always clean. But there's something about that state — living at the edge of readiness — that keeps you sharp. The body knows the drill. The mind follows. And the heart, despite the grind, still remembers why it matters.

Although the day will inevitably surprise you — an unexpected lab result, a new complaint, a curveball you couldn't anticipate — that shift, that pregame hum in your chest, is a reminder: You're stepping into work that matters. The stakes are real. The outcomes aren't abstract. And when you hit that rhythm, when the room changes over and you move seamlessly from one story to the next, it's as close to a flow state as medicine allows.

Every day starts that way for me. On the drive in, I feel the tension building. My brain is already flipping through the possibilities — who might be on the schedule, who might have been admitted overnight, what curveballs might get thrown into the day. I wonder what's in store. Will I be the calm in someone's storm? Will I get a moment to breathe? Probably not.

Still, that's the thing — this is what I do. It's what I trained for. What I chose. And even though I carry the truth that the day will take a lot from me, I also know it will give something back.

The moment I walk into the building, there's no turning back. I sit down, log in, and glance at the list. There it is. The number: 18 or 20 or 23. I don't flinch anymore. I take a deep breath, let it settle in my chest, and then I go. Because this is the work. The rhythm. The choice I've made again and again. And as much as it drains, it also sustains.

Room one. First patient. The anxiety is always there. I've done this long enough to know what's coming. The warm-up. I crack a joke. I listen closely. I examine. I think. And then — snap — I'm in the zone.

It's hard to explain to someone who's never felt it. You become both hyper-aware and completely automatic. Every movement, every question, every pause has purpose. I'm listening, responding, managing. But I'm also flowing. I'm not just present — I'm locked in.

Each patient is a puzzle, a story, a connection waiting to be made. Heart failure in one room, depression in the next, diabetes after that, and then — out of nowhere — a new cancer diagnosis. All of it in the span of an hour. And somehow, I don't lose myself in it. I find myself in it.

There's a rhythm to it, almost like music. A state of mind where time bends, where being three patients behind doesn't spark panic. I still feel calm. Focused. In control. That's the zone — not because the work is easy, and certainly not because I'm perfect, but because I've stopped resisting the current. I let it carry me. And in that current, I do my best work.

People think medicine is all data and decisions, but the real art is energy. If I bring calm, the room calms. If I bring warmth, the room opens up. That's what makes the work sustainable. That's what makes me feel whole at the end of the day, not hollowed out.

We try to keep things light in the outpatient clinic. We laugh. Humor has a way of softening the edges, reminding both patient and physician that this isn't just about lab results or blood pressure readings — it's about two people sharing space. Sometimes it's a small joke about the weather or a playful jab at how many medications I'm juggling on the screen. Other times it's a belly laugh, the kind that makes the walls of the exam room feel a little less sterile.

That laughter isn't distraction. It's medicine. It breaks tension. It opens doors. It lets patients know I'm not only interested in their lab values but in their lives. And it reminds me, too, that even on the heaviest days, joy belongs in this work.

Room after room. Case after case. Sometimes a moment stops me — bad news, tears, a subtle diagnosis that shifts everything. Yet I keep going. I stay centered. I give everything I have to each room, and somehow, I still find something left to give to the next.

Until I don't. That's how burnout sneaks in — not as one dramatic crash, but as the slow draining of a reservoir you thought was bottomless. You don't notice at first. You tell yourself you can handle it, that tomorrow will be lighter, that this is just the way it is. But day after day, the margin thins. The reset stops working. The current that once carried you forward starts to pull you under. And still, the world expects you to show up like nothing has changed.

The end of the day comes quietly. No grand finale. No standing ovation. Just the last patient, the last note, the last phone call. And then it hits me.

It's physical. My shoulders drop. My jaw unclenches. My breath slows. There's this strange sensation — like a low-grade neuropathy, energy draining down through my legs, my spine, my fingertips. A tension that's been holding me upright all day finally lets go.

It's not exhaustion, exactly. It's not burnout. It's clarity. It's the deep, satisfying exhale that only comes after you've given everything you had — and it was enough.

I don't always talk about this part: the come-down. It's not dramatic, but it's real. And it matters. It's how I carry the quiet truth that I did good work. That I showed up. That I was present. At 7 a.m. I was wound tight, a spring under pressure. But now — now I can feel my body again. I can feel myself again.

I get in my car and text Farah: I'm on my way home. Yet I'm not really back — not yet. First, I sit in silence. A few minutes to process the weight I've been carrying. To let the current ease. To come down, slowly, gently, from the zone.

The remarkable thing is, I don't dread tomorrow. That sensation, that rhythm, that zone — it's part of me now. Not addiction. Not martyrdom. Something deeper. A craft. A calling. A commitment to presence — the act of being wholly there, again and again.

People say medicine is broken, and in many ways, it is. Yet this part — the moment I step into a room, connect with another human being, and offer something of value — that remains intact. Untouched. Sacred.

In the Zone

The zone reminds me why I do this. It's where I feel most capable, most clear, most human. And when it ends — when my body finally lets go, when the tingling reminder tells me I gave everything I had — I don't regret it.

Still, even as I drive home, a question lingers: Why is this feeling bound to my workday? Why is it woven into my professional life, but not my personal one?

I don't feel this kind of clarity on a lazy Sunday. I don't find it standing in line at the grocery store. No — this is different. This is Dr. Nadelson. The version of me that exists only in the clinic. In the chaos. In the need. In the raw presence of people asking for help, trusting me with their vulnerability. In that space, I become something sharper. More focused. More alive.

It's not fake. It's not a mask. It's a version of me that only comes out when it's needed. When it matters most. And it's become part of my normal. Part of my rhythm. A familiar switch that flips as soon as I walk through those outpatient clinic doors.

That zone — that performance space — isn't unique to doctors. We all have it in different forms. Athletes. Musicians. Teachers. Parents. Anyone who shifts between identities throughout the day. Some of us visit it occasionally. Some live there. For me, I step into it daily. It's both a blessing and a weight. And the anxiety that comes with it? That tension? It isn't bad. It isn't something to fix or run from.

It's a good anxiety. Not dread. Not panic. But focus. Fuel. Passion, showing up in physical form. It's the anticipation of doing something that matters.

When I stop resisting that sensation — when I welcome it — I perform at my best. I'm sharper. I listen harder. I move with intention. I'm not coasting through the motions. I'm fully present. Fully engaged. Fully me. That's the zone. And it's where I feel most alive.

Which leaves me wondering: What exactly is perfection? Is it even real? Or is the zone itself the closest we ever come?

Each time we feel like we've arrived — reached that so-called pinnacle — something else presents itself. A new standard. A new benchmark. A new desire. We strive toward one finish line only to find another waiting ahead. It never ends. And maybe the better question isn't what is perfection, but why do we believe it exists in the first place?

Like many people, I used to think perfection was the path. Not the destination, but the compass guiding every decision. I built a mental checklist of success — what I thought I needed to accomplish to finally feel like I had made it. Not for applause or recognition, but to validate my worth. To prove I was enough.

I wanted to crush the MCAT. I definitely didn't do that.

I wanted to get into a top-tier medical school — one with prestige. That didn't happen.

I wanted to excel once I got to med school. I did pretty well.

I wanted to match into an exceptional residency program. I landed in a solid one. It gave me great training, wise mentors, and a foundation I still rely on every day. But it wasn't one of those elite institutions that makes heads turn when you say the name.

I wanted to join a respected practice. Build a meaningful career. Provide for my family. Contribute to my community. And that, I did. I'm proud of where I am.

Still, here's the truth: With every milestone I reached, the goalposts moved. Every single time. What I thought would bring arrival only brought a new standard, a new chase, a new way of feeling not quite enough.

That's the trap of perfection: It never delivers what it promises. It keeps shifting, always just beyond reach. And if you let it, it blinds you to the life you're already living, the work you're already doing, the presence you've already given.

Perfection was never the compass. Presence was. Showing up fully — not flawlessly — is what has carried me farther than any checklist ever could.

When I got into medical school, I immediately started worrying about matching. When I matched into residency, I started worrying about the kind of job I'd land. When I got the job, I thought about how to build, how to lead, how to grow.

And even now — when things are objectively going well — there's still that quiet hum beneath it all: What's next? Maybe I'll just write a book. And maybe that's the point: not another item on the checklist, not another moving goalpost, but a chance to pause, to make meaning, to tell the story instead of just chasing the next chapter.

Chasing Perfection

That's the problem with chasing perfection: It keeps moving the goalposts. You never "arrive." The target shifts. The standards rise. The bar gets higher, even after you've cleared it.

This isn't personal; it's human nature. We are wired for progress. That can be a beautiful thing. It drives innovation, growth, and evolution. Yet it also means we're prone to dissatisfaction, even amid success. We normalize our achievements so quickly that they barely register as victories before we're on to the next challenge.

And in medicine, this mindset is deeply embedded. The training path itself conditions us to believe that satisfaction is always deferred. First, do well in college. Then ace the MCAT. Then survive med school. Then match. Then finish training. Then get a job. Then get a better job. Then start earning. Then start leading. Then publish. Then teach. Then what?

We don't leave room to celebrate the wins. We're too busy bracing for the next exam, the next evaluation, the next promotion, the next responsibility. It's a system built on delayed gratification — and the delay never seems to end.

At some point, we have to ask: What are we chasing? Is it prestige? Praise? Security? Purpose? And is there ever a moment when we stop long enough to believe that we are already enough?

For me, that shift came slowly. Not in the big milestones, but in the quieter ones. A patient's trust. A colleague's gratitude. My kids running to the door when I walk in at night. Those aren't boxes to check; they're reminders that the point was never perfection, it was presence.

I may never silence that voice asking what's next? But I've learned that "enough" isn't somewhere down the road. It's here, in the work I get to do, the people I get to love, and the moments I choose to notice before they pass me by.

I don't think we talk about this enough — how easy it is to feel like we're underperforming, even when we're thriving. How the comparison game creeps in through each crack, whispering that someone else is doing it better. How we carry this unspoken belief that there's some ideal version of ourselves we haven't reached but should have by now.

The idea of having it all together is seductive. But perfection is a mirage, a horizon line that shifts the closer we get. Chase it long enough, and it will steal more than it gives. It robs us of joy. Of presence. Of peace.

So what's the alternative? For me, it's shifting the metric. Measuring success not by arbitrary benchmarks or external applause, but by something more grounded: alignment.

Am I doing work that reflects my values?

Am I growing in ways that feel authentic to who I am?

Am I showing up for my family, my colleagues, my patients?

Am I using my strengths to make a difference?

Am I curious? Still honest? Still trying?

If the answer is yes, then I'm where I need to be.

That doesn't mean I've stopped setting goals. I have ambition. I push myself. But I'm more mindful now of why I'm pushing. Is it out of inspiration or insecurity? Am I chasing impact or validation?

And when I find myself shifting the goalposts again, I try to pause. Reflect. Take inventory of how far I've come. For the truth is, I already surpassed the version of me that once dreamed of being here.

When I was younger, I thought the destination was everything. Now I carry the truth: It's about the journey. The people. The growth. The quiet pride that comes from knowing you showed up again and again. Even when it was hard — especially when it was hard.

And if you ask me now what success means, I won't point to degrees or titles or institutions. I'll point to effort. Integrity. Consistency. I'll point to the mornings I wake up grounded in purpose. To the evenings I come home and look at my kids and feel peace. To the spaces in between — the ones no résumé ever captures — where I carry the truth that I've lived fully and honestly.

Moving goalposts don't have to define us; they're part of the process. Yet they don't have to steal the joy of where we are now. Perfection may be a myth, but being present — that's real. And that's enough for me.

The Need to Step Away

Sometimes what you need most isn't more effort, but less. A breath. A pause. A moment to recalibrate. Not every problem is solved by motion. Not every challenge demands more pushing, more striving. Sometimes the most profound shift comes when you stop long enough to breathe.

We juggle expectations, schedules, responsibilities. And in the midst of that, it's easy to forget that we are not machines. We're human. We get tired. We break down. And yet, we rarely give ourselves permission to pause. We treat rest like a reward instead of a requirement. We view time off as weakness, or worse: a luxury. If there's one thing I have come to understand over the years, both as a doctor and as a human being, it's this: We move fast. We push through. We have to pause — on purpose. Not because we've earned it. Not because everything is fine. But because our humanity depends on it.

We live in a culture that idolizes productivity. We measure our worth in output, in how much we can carry without crumbling. We celebrate endurance, hustle, grit. Rarely do we celebrate wisdom — the wisdom to stop before we break. The wisdom to say, "This moment matters, and I don't need to be everything to everyone right now."

It's not just air filling your lungs; it's clarity returning to your mind. Stillness pushing back against the storm. Presence.

You remember who you are. Where you are. What matters. It's a reset. A reframe.

And often, that reset doesn't come in the middle of your inbox. It doesn't come while running room to room, checking boxes, chasing deadlines. Sometimes, the most important thing you can do — for yourself, your patients, your family — is to step away. Sometimes, the deep breath you need isn't a literal breath. It's a break. A vacation. A change of scenery. A physical and mental pause from the world you spend every day trying to manage.

Not the trip you half-plan and cancel. Not the one you keep promising you'll take someday. Take the real vacation — the one where your phone is off, your inbox stays closed, and your spirit is finally given permission to rise again. Travel somewhere new. Or stay close to home and do something that fills your soul.

Sleep in. Read. Walk with your kids. Breathe. It's not about escape. It's about rhythm. Cycles. Perspective.

You can't always be "on." So many of us struggle with this — especially in medicine. We become so entangled in our roles that stepping away feels impossible, even irresponsible. We tell ourselves the system needs us. That patients need us. That things will fall apart without us.

Still, here's the truth: Things fall apart within us when we never step away.

We don't talk about that part. We talk about duty. About showing up. About being reliable, dedicated, irreplaceable. And while those values matter, they mean little if you become a shell of the person who once embodied them.

Even a short pause can change your trajectory. Even a small vacation can realign your perspective. Even a weekend with your family — fully present, unplugged — can restore parts of you that felt permanently depleted.

Rest is not the opposite of responsibility. It's what allows you to carry responsibility without losing yourself to it. When you take that step back — when you finally exhale — you often see your world differently. You gain distance. You gain clarity. What felt urgent may no longer feel important. What felt insurmountable may suddenly seem manageable. And what felt like the end of you? Maybe it's not the end at all. Maybe it's the beginning of something else.

You remember that your life isn't made up of tasks and charts and diagnoses. It's made up of people. Moments. Joy. Breath. And if you think about who will be beside you when the work slows down — when the job titles fade and the accolades are forgotten — it won't be the system. It will be the people you love. The ones you've known the longest. The ones who see you even when you don't say a word.

They're the ones who know when you're not okay. Who sense your stress before you speak it. Who drop everything the second they know you need them. That kind of support can't be faked. It's not built overnight. It's built in dinners shared, in vacations taken, in evenings where nothing "productive" happens except being together.

So why do we keep putting those moments off?

We delay them for the future, as if we're guaranteed time. As if the perfect window will eventually open, and then we'll rest. Then we'll take the trip. Then we'll make the call. Sadly, life doesn't work that way. The window doesn't open; you have to carve it out.

This isn't about burnout prevention; it's about survival. About preservation. About knowing when you need to pull over before you crash.

As physicians, we're taught how to triage emergencies. We know when a patient needs oxygen, fluids, or intervention. We're not trained to recognize our own vital signs. We normalize the slow bleed. The chronic fatigue. The creeping cynicism. We accept it as part of the job, part of the sacrifice.

What if it's not? The thought of that creeping feeling isn't the cost of doing medicine, but a sign that something needs to change. Maybe the most courageous thing you can do isn't to work through it; maybe it's stepping away. Maybe it's saying, "I'm not okay. And I need to rest before I become unrecognizable to myself."

That's not weakness. That's wisdom. That's strength. Not because you're failing, but because you're worth saving before you fall apart.

You don't need to be everything to everyone. You need to be you: grounded, present, human. And sometimes, finding your way back to that version of yourself starts with something simple.

Never forget: You are replaceable. The system will keep moving. The inbox will keep filling. The schedule will keep spinning. But in the exam room — on that stage where knowledge collides with humanity — something different happens. That space cannot be replaced. It belongs to you and the person sitting across from you.

In that room, medicine becomes less about answers and more about presence. Less about perfection and more about connection. Less about fixing and more about being.

That is where the work is sacred. That is where the meaning lives.

That is why we stay.

PART III

The System and the Strain

This is where we cross the threshold into the exam room. Here, knowledge meets humanity and lessons are no longer abstract. They breathe, they speak, they stay with you. The real practice of medicine is not written in textbooks; it is written in the quiet act of showing up. In the exam room, answers matter — but presence is what changes lives.

As doctors, we don't practice medicine in a vacuum. We navigate a system that often feels chaotic, bureaucratic, and broken. We face pressures not in our outpatient clinics, but in the contracts, politics, and policies that shape how we work. In an environment where the practice of medicine collides with modern healthcare's complexity. Artificial intelligence is transforming industries, streamlining workflows, and reshaping how we interact with the world. From Silicon Valley to hospital residency hallways, the race is on for speed, precision, and an edge. Medicine is not immune to this movement, yet it is unique in what's at stake.

AI technology transcribes our notes and translates our conversations. It sifts through labs, images, and patient data with breathtaking speed. It can help predict outcomes, flag patterns, and reduce human error.

For that, we should be grateful. Yet technology is a tool, not a healer.

I've practiced long enough to witness medicine's evolution. I've seen paper charts give way to digital dashboards. I've seen algorithms outperform human eyes in detecting certain conditions, but I've also seen something AI can't do — and likely never will.

It can't comfort a grieving spouse. It can't hear the fear behind a patient's silence. It can't look someone in the eye and say, "You're going to be okay," with the weight of lived experience behind it.

What AI offers is information. What humans offer is interpretation. Meaning. Connection.

We also must acknowledge the dangers of over reliance. People often go all in on new technology, hoping it holds all the answers. AI doesn't deliver certainty; it delivers possibilities. It casts a wide net. It may offer hundreds of potential diagnoses, many of which are irrelevant, misleading, or even frightening.

And that leads to something we don't talk about enough: the emotional consequences of digital misdiagnosis.

A patient Googles their symptoms and spirals. A headache becomes a brain tumor. Stomach pain becomes cancer. A harmless symptom becomes a life-altering fear. Suddenly, the patient isn't dealing with discomfort; they're battling anxiety, panic, and worst-case-scenario thinking.

Faster isn't always better. Information at your fingertips is only helpful if you understand how to interpret it through a human lens. Just because something is accessible doesn't make it accurate. Being fast doesn't make it right. There's no algorithm for nuance. No chatbot that can replicate context. No app that can replace empathy.

And even beyond empathy, let's not forget practicality. Can AI understand your family dynamics? Does it know your spouse? Your kids? Your stressors? Your support system? Can it recommend local specialists or community resources based not on credentials, but on character?

That's not data; that's discernment, judgment, humanity.

AI can't customize advice for each unique individual. It can't blend science with experience, or evidence with emotion. That's where physicians step in — not just as diagnosticians, but as guides.

And this truth extends far beyond the exam room. Think about calling your insurance company or your airline. You're met with a chatbot, a voice prompt, a loop. What do most people do? They press "0." They ask for a person. Why? Because we don't just want answers. We want clarity. We want someone who understands our question — and our context.

AI is powerful for basic information. But when it comes to solving real problems, what matters most is human contact.

Medicine is no different. At its core, it is — and always will be — human. I may be in the minority, but I believe that truth will never change. People prefer to speak with a real person — whether disputing a phone bill, managing a credit card balance, or deciding where to invest their savings. That's not something we trust to a chatbot. We want a voice. We want understanding. We want confidence that the advice applies to us.

Yes, there is a place for artificial intelligence. It has value, and even brilliance. But it cannot replace the judgment, empathy, and trust required to truly heal. That is a line we cannot cross — and one developers and technologists must take seriously.

AI is a powerful utility. But it is not, and never will be, a substitute for human connection. So no, AI will not remove the human from medicine. Not unless we let it.

When I became chair of the Department of Internal Medicine at our multispecialty outpatient clinic in Northeast Georgia — part of the Northside Hospital system — I didn't feel any different. There was no spotlight. No big announcement. No internal shift in how I saw myself. My routine stayed the same: I woke up early, saw patients, and spent my days trying to help people feel better, listened to, and understood. My title at the clinic may have changed, but to my patients, I was still just Dr. Nadelson. Leadership didn't change who I was. It gave me a new kind of responsibility.

We're the largest department in our practice, and we continue to grow. I've had the opportunity to be a part of that growth — interviewing new physicians, collaborating on department goals, and helping to shape the kind of team I'd want to work in myself. I've never seen leadership as a platform for control. If anything, I believe the best leaders are the ones who get out of the way.

I've never wanted to micromanage anyone. We're professionals. Adults. Doctors, PAs, NPs, MAs — we all bring our own strengths and pressures, both inside and outside the outpatient clinic. Some of us are parents. Some are caregivers. Some are fighting silent battles no one knows about. I try never to forget that. My job isn't to dictate. My job is to create an environment where people can thrive. That's why I focus on building trust, not power.

When new clinicians join our team, I tell them this is their time to shine. I don't want to interfere with how they practice. I'm here to support them, not monitor them. If I've done my job right, they'll never feel like they're being watched; they'll feel like they're being backed.

This philosophy stems from my own journey in medicine. Like many physicians, I've been on the receiving end of systems that didn't always feel supportive. Systems where burnout simmered beneath the surface. Where hierarchy stifled collaboration. I knew if I ever found myself in a leadership role, I'd want to do things differently.

So I lead with humility. I lead like a colleague, not a commander. I don't need to be liked — but I am liked, I think, because I don't pretend to be anything I'm not. I'm not chasing prestige. I'm not interested in office politics. I don't need to be the loudest voice in the room. My allegiance is, and always has been, to the patients — and to the people who care for them.

That's where I find meaning. They allow me to be an outpatient clinician first. They trust me to care for my team and my department without constantly pulling me away from the bedside. That kind of respect is rare, and it allows me to stay grounded in the work I love most.

Some people assume that leadership is isolating, that it must be lonely at the top. I've never felt that. I owe that in large part to the administration I work with. Having to balance what's best for one individual with what's best for the department — these aren't always easy calls to make. Leadership isn't about being perfect; it's about being steady. It's about being honest. It's about remembering that you don't have to know everything, but you do have to listen.

There are moments when difficult decisions land on your shoulders. Times when colleagues look to you for clarity when you don't have all the answers.

I listen when someone needs help managing their workload. I listen when there's tension between colleagues. I listen when someone's feeling overwhelmed and needs to talk. Leadership, at its core, is about presence. You don't always have to fix things. Sometimes, being there is enough.

The way we show up for one another. The way we cover for someone without making them feel guilty for asking. A healthy department isn't an accident; it takes intention. It takes reinforcement. It takes someone quietly paying attention, even when everything seems fine on the surface.

It's also about protecting the culture of the department — something that's harder to define, but easy to feel. It's in the way we talk to each other. That's what I try to do, and I love that responsibility. Not because it feeds my ego, but because it feeds my purpose.

And yet, through all of this, I don't see myself as "the leader." I see myself as one of the many. I carry my own patient panel. I get behind on my inbox. I share the same frustrations, joys, and fatigue as other outpatient clinicians in our group. That connection keeps me real. It keeps me grounded. Titles come and go. Roles shift. But who you are in the exam room — the one they trust — that sticks with you. That's the kind of leadership I value. The kind that doesn't need recognition to be real. Leadership doesn't have to be loud. It doesn't have to be lonely, and it doesn't have to pull you away from what you love.

Sometimes, the strongest form of leadership is the quiet kind — the kind that supports more than it directs, listens more than it speaks, and elevates others without needing the credit. That's the kind I believe in. That's the kind I try to live.

Back to Your Why

From the moment I step into the outpatient clinic, the deluge begins: messages, lab results, abnormal vitals, staff questions, urgent follow-ups. It's unending. Everyone wants answers, and they want them now. The volume of tasks isn't high — it's personal. Each one represents a life. A fear. A hope.

Medicine is not demanding; it's relentless. It's a profession of ceaseless expectation, where the needs of others constantly override your own. There have been moments — many, if I'm honest — when walking away felt like a real option. Not because I don't care, but because I care so much that it hurts.

Burnout is real. It's not a buzzword. It's a slow unraveling. It creeps in quietly — first as fatigue, then as irritation, then as cynicism. And before you know it, you're asking questions you never thought you'd raise: Can I keep doing this? Should I? What would life look like if I walked away from medicine?

So why didn't I? I've built something here: relationships, trust, continuity. I'm the doctor that people rely on, not for prescriptions or diagnoses, but for guidance, for reassurance, for presence — being wholly there. That kind of trust doesn't come easily, and it doesn't come often. I hold it tightly.

Many of my patients see me as one of the most stable figures in their lives. They bring me their uncertainty, their pain, and sometimes, the need to be seen. That matters to me. That keeps me grounded.

Stress doesn't deter me anymore; it motivates me. It sharpens my focus. It reminds me that I'm growing. I'm learning, every single day, not about medicine, but about people. About what makes them tick. About what they need when they're vulnerable. About how to be real with them when things fall apart.

When I think about leaving, I think about my children. I think about the example I want to set — not about career, but about grit. About purpose. About the kind of life worth living. And it's always changing.

That's one of the hardest parts. Just when you get your bearings. Something shifts: new regulations, new systems, new expectations. Sometimes it's for the better. Sometimes, it feels like change for the sake of change. And as physicians, we're expected to adapt on the fly, to run at full speed while rewriting the playbook in real time.

COVID was the clearest example. It didn't just change how we practiced — it upended what it even meant to be a doctor.

Telemedicine overnight. Clinics shut down. New safety protocols. PPE shortages. Fear. Uncertainty. Grief. Everything we thought was stable had to be reinvented. There was no time to hesitate. We had to adapt — fast. And we did. We adapted because we had to. It wasn't easy. But that's what we do.

These shifts in medicine are deeply personal. They affect how we care, how we connect, and how we carry the weight of this work. Every change ripples through the patient experience and into our own lives. We are doctors and humans. Always both. And staying in this field means accepting that reality. The identity, the role, the sacrifice — it all evolves, just as we do.

Sure, medicine has changed. The prestige isn't the same. The workload is heavier. The compensation often doesn't match the sacrifice. Fewer medical students are choosing primary care or internal medicine. The pipeline is thinning. The system is stressed, and it's stressing us out with it.

I don't work for the system. I work for the patient who brings me a teacup from her travels because she remembered something I once said in passing. I work for the family who calls me first when their father is in crisis. I work for the aspiring doctor who watches me manage chaos with calm and says, "I want to learn to be like that."

Medicine is broken in many ways. We all know that, yet the meaning in medicine? That's intact. You have to dig a little deeper to find it sometimes.

Go back to your first white coat ceremony. To the patient who first called you "doctor." To the moment you made someone feel safe by being in the room. To any physician reading this who's feeling frayed at the edges, I won't pretend to have the answers, but I will say this: Go back to your "why." Go back to the moment you first filled out your medical school application, when the dream felt pure and the mission clear.

Burnout tries to steal that from you. Don't let it.

Sometimes the answer isn't to walk away. Sometimes it's to walk back in with clearer boundaries, better support, and a stronger sense of self. You may not be able to fix the system. But you can reclaim your place in it. For me, staying wasn't about obligation; it was about alignment. This is the life I want. I get to be a husband, a father, a physician, and a human being — all in one life. Not always in perfect balance, but in honest effort.

That's enough. That's why I stayed.

To the staff. To the nurses. It's woven into the fabric of every hallway and exam room. It pulses in the unspoken silence after a difficult diagnosis, the weight we carry after a code blue, the fear we try to suppress when a case doesn't go the way we hoped.

We often think of it as something we treat in others — patients who walk through the door with anxiety, depression, trauma, grief. And it is. Yet it also belongs to us. To the doctors.

The Reality of Burnout

This profession demands emotional energy at all times. We deal with joy, anger, despair — often within the same hour. One moment, we're delivering good news, and the next, we're walking into a room where someone's world is about to fall apart. You never quite know what's waiting behind the next door.

There are moments we want to forget but can't. There's no off switch. Even after we clock out, the weight comes home with us. We sit at the dinner table still thinking about the labs we reviewed, the scan we're worried about, the note we forgot to chart. We wake in the middle of the night replaying a conversation, wondering if we missed something. There are stories we hear that we wish we hadn't. Cases that replay in our minds without warning.

This isn't something we're trained for in medical school. There's no textbook chapter on carrying the emotional weight of medicine. And yet, we don't talk about it. Not in residency. Not during morning rounds. Not in the elevator ride between patients.

Depression is real. Burnout is real. The numbers are staggering: More than one in four physicians screen positive for depression. One in 10 have contemplated suicide. Suicide rates among physicians are more than double those of the general population for women, and 70% higher for men. According to the American Medical Association and Medscape's 2024 report on physician burnout, nearly 53% of doctors report feeling burned out.

Those numbers aren't sobering — they're horrifying. Behind each number is a physician — someone who once dreamed of making a difference, now wondering if they can keep going. A colleague, a friend, a parent, a mentor.

We talk about resilience, but too often we confuse it with silence. We push forward, chart after chart, day after day, even as the weight grows heavier. And when physicians break, we act as if it's an anomaly — when in truth, it is everywhere around us.

These numbers are not statistics to memorize. They are warnings. They are stories unfinished. And they are a call to make medicine safer — not just for patients, but for those who provide the care.

Behind every statistic is a doctor who once dreamed of helping others — now silently struggling to survive their own battles. These aren't abstract figures; they're our colleagues, our friends, sometimes ourselves.

And the tragedy is not only the loss of life, but the silence that surrounds it. We don't talk about it enough. We don't prepare physicians for the emotional toll of medicine. And too often, we allow the stigma of vulnerability to keep us quiet when we most need to speak.

Maybe that's why the numbers are so staggering. Medicine is a breeding ground for anxiety. The fear of failure is constant. The fear of making a mistake, of letting someone down — whether a patient, a colleague, a staff member, or your own family — is always there.

That pit in your stomach isn't rare; it's a familiar companion. Every decision is laced with consequence. Every order. Every diagnosis. Every word. Each one carries weight. And yet, we're expected to hold it all together. We're expected to be composed. Compassionate. Sharp. Tireless. On point. Every. Single. Day.

We live with a deep, underlying worry that everything could change at any moment. Life feels fine — until it's not. The detour comes suddenly. A medical error. A malpractice case. A personal crisis. A health scare of our own. A patient we couldn't help. We know how fragile life is. We see it daily. That knowledge doesn't free us — it haunts us.

Strength Amid Silence

Physicians are often perceived as resilient, almost superhuman. The reality is, we're human. We're not immune to the weight of the work. We're not unaffected by the tears we see, the deaths we witness, the mistakes we agonize over. We don't always bounce back. We carry these things in silence. The irony is that in a profession centered around health, mental health among doctors is often the most neglected.

There's the fear of stigma — the worry that if we admit we're struggling, we'll be seen as weak, unstable, or unfit to practice.

A 2023 study published in *JAMA* found that nearly 40% of physicians avoid seeking mental health treatment out of fear it will negatively impact their licensure or career. I'd argue the real number is even higher.

The unspoken truth is that many of us have quietly skipped therapy, avoided medication, or hidden our struggles — not because we didn't need help, but because we feared the consequences of being honest.

In medicine, strength is often defined as endurance, as the ability to keep going no matter the cost. But that definition is broken. Endurance without support isn't resilience — it's erosion. Until we can speak openly about our mental health without fear of losing our licenses, our positions, or the trust of our peers, the silence will persist. And that silence costs lives — ours.

There's the lack of time, the lack of access, the lack of space to be vulnerable. Mostly, there's the silence. For where are we supposed to talk about it? Not with our patients — that would be unprofessional. They're not there for us. We're there for them. Not always with our families — it's hard to translate the things we see and feel into words that make sense to someone who hasn't been inside this world. Not always with our colleagues — we're all performing the same act: stable, competent, always okay.

Beneath the coat and the clicks, many of us are not okay. Behind the smile, some of us are barely holding it together. We say "I'm fine" because it's easier than explaining the weight we carry. Easier than admitting the burnout. Easier than confronting the fear that asking for help might label us as broken. We're not broken. We're human. Mental health in medicine isn't a side conversation. It's *the* conversation.

We need to normalize therapy, peer support, mental health days. We need to change licensure questions that penalize physicians for getting the help they need. We need to remind each other — and ourselves — that struggling doesn't make you a bad doctor; it makes you a real one. We need to talk about it more openly — in training, in outpatient clinics, in hospitals. We need systems that support doctors not as outpatient clinicians but as people.

Until then, many of us will continue to carry our burdens quietly. We'll nod and smile through the day while anxiety brews underneath. We'll show up for others while trying not to fall apart ourselves.

Maybe the most healing thing we can do — for ourselves and for each other — is to break that silence.

Pivot, Adapt, Survive

The essence of medicine is human, not absolute. There was no clear answer, yet there was one undeniable truth: I could not keep going the way I was. I was running on empty. Something needed to change.

I reassessed my routines. I started sleeping better, eating better, and being more honest with myself. I asked for help instead of pretending I could do it all. I spent more time reviewing cases, not to impress anyone, but to regain confidence in my own thinking. I adapted my mindset — not because it was easy, but because I had to.

I realized that pivot is not weakness; it is wisdom. It is not about giving up; it is about giving yourself permission to grow in a different direction. Too often, we frame change as quitting. We say someone "gave up" or "walked away" when they veer off the expected path, yet life is not linear. Pivot is responding to reality with flexibility and intention. It is one of the most important skills we can develop — not as professionals, but as people.

When I first imagined being a doctor, I pictured the traditional model: The same physician who saw you in the office would be the one to check on you in the hospital. That continuity carried a certain comfort: one doctor, one relationship, one thread of care that followed you through every stage.

That world has changed. Today, my work is strictly outpatient. I see my patients in the clinic, manage their chronic conditions, adjust their medications, and try to keep them well. But when one of them ends up in the hospital, the care transfers to a hospitalist team: physicians whose focus is entirely on inpatient medicine. They do the important work of stabilizing, admitting, and treating acute illness, while I remain on the outside, waiting to pick things back up when my patient is discharged.

Alongside this shift, hybrid models have emerged. Practices now weave together traditional in-person visits with telehealth and digital tools, giving patients both the depth of face-to-face care and the ease of remote access.

And then there are the practices that have gone fully virtual. Some companies never see patients in person at all. Everything — consultations, prescriptions, follow-ups — happens through a screen. For certain conditions and certain patients, it works. For others, it leaves something missing.

Specialists adapt in their own ways. Some remain fully embedded in the hospital. Others split their time — office hours on one side, procedures or inpatient consults on the other. Every branch of medicine seems to be carving its own path.

If I've learned anything, it's that medicine never sits still. The models are always shifting, reshaping themselves around technology, patient needs, and the realities of the system. At first it felt strange, even unsettling, to let go of that traditional role where one doctor followed a patient everywhere. But I've come to see it as the natural rhythm of this profession. We pivot. We adapt. We find new ways to show up.

And the truth is, this constant evolution isn't unique to medicine — it's simply how the world works.

When COVID-19 swept through our lives, we pivoted overnight. Telemedicine, once an afterthought, became the lifeline of healthcare. We adapted from packed waiting rooms to remote care. From handshakes and heart-to-hearts in exam rooms to Zoom visits and pixelated expressions. From routine care to crisis management.

And yet, we did not stop showing up. We adapted. We changed our workflows. We developed new safety protocols. We treated patients in PPE that left marks on our faces and fatigue in our bones. We adapted to new treatment algorithms, new billing systems, new staffing shortages — and through it all, we kept going.

We pivot when insurance rewrites the rules of billing. We pivot when Medicare adds new regulations. We pivot when staffing runs short, when burnout creeps in, when the weight of the system forces us to recalibrate — not only how we care for others, but how we care for ourselves.

As parents, we pivot every day. What works for one does not always work for another. One child needs structure; the other needs freedom. One child responds to a firm tone; the other needs gentleness. We adapt. We try again.

In relationships, we pivot, too. We learn to listen more and speak less. We learn when to lean in and when to give space. We evolve with our partners, our friends, our families. Relationships grow because we are willing to shift — not because we got it right the first time.

And even in the smallest, most mundane moments, pivot is a quiet kind of power.

You are mid-conversation, and something does not land the way you hoped — pivot.

You try a new recipe and it falls flat — pivot.

You start a workout routine and injure your knee — pivot.

You feel lost, stuck, uncertain — pause, reflect, adapt, and pivot.

Being flexible, malleable, is not a liability. It is a strength. The ability to adapt, to reassess, to change course when needed — that is how we survive. That is how we succeed.

It is also how we stay in alignment with who we are. For sometimes, staying the course is not bravery — it is stubbornness, and pivot is not failure — it is growth. You can pivot without shame. You can pivot a thousand times in one lifetime. Each turn is a declaration: I am paying attention. I am not giving up. I am choosing a new path forward.

That is what I want to teach my kids. That is what I want my patients to feel when they're scared to make a change. That's what I remind myself when life doesn't go as planned.

We all fall. We all doubt. Yet the people who go far — the ones who truly grow — are the ones who learn to pivot, again and again.

So the next time you hit a wall, don't quit. Stop. Breathe. Reflect. Ask yourself what's working, what's not, and what needs to shift. Because sometimes the bravest move isn't staying the course — it's daring to change it.

Changing a Mindset

Medicine is a career — not a lifelong vow of self-sacrifice. Yes, for some, medicine may feel like a calling. Yet, choosing to become a physician is not a binding contract to make it your entire identity forever. Times have changed; our mindset must, too.

It is not a betrayal of the profession to work part-time, seek better balance, or transition into leadership, education, innovation, or non-outpatient clinical roles. Too often, these choices are viewed as abandonment rather than evolution.

We must reject the outdated belief that one must devote every waking moment to outpatient clinical practice in order to be "worthy" of the MD title. This mindset is not only inaccurate, it's harmful. It alienates future doctors, burns out current ones, and distorts what this profession can and should be.

Medicine is a job — yes, an incredibly meaningful one — but like any profession, it must allow space for growth, change, and personal reinvention. To tell young people that medicine demands a full-throttle, lifelong commitment or nothing at all is, frankly, career malpractice.

Supporting physicians means understanding that how one chooses to practice does not determine if they matter. We need a culture that embraces flexibility, encourages humanity, and values all forms of contribution — outpatient clinical and beyond.

After a decade in practice, I have yet to meet a physician who willingly endured four years of college, four years of medical school, and at least three years of residency or fellowship to gain a title. The idea that young people would choose a path marked by enormous debt, personal sacrifice, and years of delayed gratification for prestige alone is implausible at best — and insulting at worst.

If you want to understand what's driving physicians out of outpatient clinical roles, ask those of us doing the work. We're not difficult to reach. Most of us are eager to share our insights and contribute to meaningful change.

The majority of physicians are not disillusioned with medicine. We are deeply committed to our patients. We are proud of the care we provide. What discourages us is not the work itself — it's the system around it: the relentless administrative burdens, the outdated technologies, the regulatory red tape — all of which pull us further from the bedside and away from the people we're here to help.

The path forward begins with support. And that support starts with how we view each other. Because the truth is, medicine isn't a solo act. It has never been. It is, and always will be, a team effort.

I am proud to be a physician. I'm honored to care for an extraordinary patient community. But I also believe that supporting this profession means letting go of rigid, antiquated expectations about what a physician "should" look like.

These are not minor frustrations. They are structural problems that erode morale and reduce the time we can spend with patients. They deserve serious attention from policymakers, hospital residency leaders, and the public.

We must stop shaming those who seek a healthier, more sustainable path within or adjacent to medicine. We must challenge the idea that outpatient clinical intensity is the only marker of impact. And above all, we must listen to the doctors who are showing up every day, even as the system grows heavier on their shoulders.

It's time to lead better, support better, and build a medical culture rooted in empathy, flexibility, and truth. Not for physicians — but for the patients we all serve.

We Can't and Don't Do It Alone

There's a common misconception in medicine: that the doctor is the centerpiece, the singular figure of importance. Let me be clear: Nothing in my day happens without my team.

My first team is my home team. My wife and kids are the foundation of everything I do. They are my why. They remind me what matters most. Their love gives me purpose, their support gives me strength, and their belief in me keeps me moving forward — even on the hardest days. They sacrifice so I can serve others. They don't wear white coats, but they make my work possible.

They never clock out. They love me unconditionally. They understand the emotional toll. They wait patiently when I'm running behind, pick up the slack when I'm overwhelmed, and welcome me back when I've given all I had to give. Their support is quiet, steady, and constant. And it's everything.

And then there's my outpatient clinical team — the heartbeat of my practice. They anticipate needs before I speak them. They know how I think, how I work, and what I expect — not because they have to, but because they care. My two medical assistants are nothing short of exceptional. They manage time, handle patient concerns, put out fires, and calm storms before they reach my door. They don't support me; they elevate me.

I work alongside a group of professionals who do more than keep the wheels turning. They bring order to chaos. Behind every smooth appointment, every timely result, every refilled prescription, there's a team making it happen. Scheduling, lab orders, insurance battles, prior authorizations, medication issues, patient messages — the never-ending logistics that rarely get noticed … unless something goes wrong. Yet day after day, my team gets it right.

When even one piece falters, the whole system feels it. It's like dominoes — one falls, and the rest are right behind. A delayed lab, a missed call, an insurance denial — each small disruption sets off a chain reaction that ripples through the clinic.

Other times it feels like musical chairs — constantly shifting, squeezing in, trying to make space for every patient before the music stops and the clinic lights go out. There's never quite enough time, never quite enough seats, but somehow, we keep moving.

That's why medicine can never be mistaken for a solo act. It isn't one person carrying the load, but a coordinated effort. It's a symphony — every role, every note, every rhythm working together. And when each part is played well, the result is harmony. Every note matters.

A practice isn't built on one person; it's built on people who show up early, stay late, adapt on the fly, and care deeply — even when no one's watching. They answer phones with patience. Greet patients with kindness. Draw blood, send referrals, fix errors, solve problems — and rarely get the credit they deserve.

Yes, I make the final clinical decisions. But I don't manage every detail of the day. I don't field every message, complete every form, or troubleshoot every glitch. I depend on the people around me. I lean on their expertise, their resilience, their commitment. And I trust them because they earn that trust every single day.

My medicals assistants are more than employees; they're my work family. I know their stories, and they know mine. We celebrate victories together and push through the rough days side by side. They carry the weight of this practice as much as I do — sometimes more.

We're in the business of healing — of lifting others when they need us most. Yet no one can do it alone. It takes a team to carry the weight, to share the mission, to make all of this possible. And I couldn't be more grateful to have mine.

Succeeding Within the System

To survive the system, you have to learn how to move within it. And sometimes, the smartest move is the quietest one.

In a world obsessed with broadcasting every step, I've come to understand the value of doing the opposite. I plan in silence. I move in stealth.

Not because I'm secretive, but because I'm strategic. Whether you're negotiating a contract, considering a career pivot, or quietly building something new, keeping your vision close to the chest can be one of your greatest advantages.

Ideas need time to grow. Expose them too early, and they invite judgment, pressure, and unrealistic expectations. I've seen it across industries, but especially in medicine, where perception often overshadows potential.

Take contract negotiations. You're not discussing a salary; you're defining your value. Oversharing too soon gives away leverage. When the other party knows your fallback plan, financial ceiling, or personal limits, the conversation shifts in their favor. That's why preparation matters. Show up with data, not desperation. Know your worth. Do your research. Protect your bottom line. Because no matter how collegial the tone may seem, the other side is negotiating for themselves, not for you.

The same holds true when buying a home, selling a business, or making any other major financial decision. Just because you can spend more doesn't mean you should. Because you've built something valuable doesn't mean the world needs access to your internal metrics or long-term goals.

Transparency is often mistaken for openness. Yet in negotiations, it's often exposure, and exposure, when premature, weakens your position. In medicine, strategic silence is often undervalued. We equate honesty with full disclosure, but that's not always wise.

Patients switch doctors for convenience. Physicians leave jobs for better pay or better balance. Colleagues cheer you on — until you become their competition. It's not cynical; it's real. Everyone has their own motives, their own needs, their own bottom line. That doesn't make people bad; it makes them human. Still, it also means we have to protect what's ours: our energy, our ideas, our plans.

Some of the most meaningful things I've built — professionally and personally — happened quietly. No fanfare. No announcements. I have come to understand that silence isn't weakness; it's discipline. In a world full of noise, the quiet ones often build the loudest results.

So when people ask what I'm working on, I stay intentionally vague — not to withhold, but to protect myself, my aspirations, and my interests. Focused. Disciplined. Deliberate.

Not every move needs a microphone. Not every plan needs an audience. Sometimes the best way to win — is to build quietly. To plan in stealth. And even with strategy and silence, one more thing is required: thick skin.

One of the hardest truths in medicine isn't medical at all: it's learning how to deal with people: the ones who appreciate you, the ones who attack you, the ones who smile and nod, the ones who say things that are offensive, personal, or flat-out inappropriate. Sometimes it's in the exam room. Sometimes it's a phone call. Sometimes it's a family member who needs someone to blame.

One complaint would send me into a spiral.

I'd come home angry, vent to my wife, and question whether I was even good at this. She'd tell me, "Let it go." Still I couldn't. It felt like a direct shot at my character. My competence. My soul. It hurt. Because medicine is personal.

Developing Thick Skin

We put so much of ourselves into the work — our time, our energy, our identity. So when someone lashes out or makes a harsh comment, it's hard not to feel like they're lashing out at you as a person. That's where thick skin comes in. The kind you build — patient by patient, year after year.

And let me be clear: Thick skin doesn't mean you stop caring. It doesn't mean you ignore feedback or deflect accountability. It means you learn to separate someone's reaction from your reality. Because you'll meet people at their worst — grieving, scared, angry, confused. They won't always say the right thing. They won't always be fair.

The online doctor reviews? Of course we read them. Sometimes, they're the only feedback we get beyond a brief conversation in the exam room.

These days, there are platforms that rate everything: whether the physician washed their hands, whether the waiting room smelled nice, whether the nurse smiled. And honestly? Transparency isn't the problem. Patients should be able to share their experience. Still, there's something missing: perspective.

A five-star rating rarely tells the full story. Neither does a one-star complaint. Maybe I was running behind because I had just spent an extra 30 minutes with another patient who got bad news. Maybe the waiting room felt crowded because half the staff had called out sick and the rest of the team was working double. Maybe the nurse didn't smile because she had just come from a room where someone's loved one had died.

None of that context makes the patient's experience less real. But it does make it incomplete. What reviews can't capture is the tension we live in every day: balancing thorough care with time pressure, compassion with exhaustion, presence with paperwork. Patients see the outcome. They rarely see the circumstances.

So yes, we read the reviews. We learn from them when we can. But if you really want to understand a physician, look beyond the stars. Look at the moments that don't make it into a comment box — the moments where medicine is messy, human, and rarely reducible to a score.

There's no second side to the story. And even worse — we can't respond. Publicly defending ourselves can come across as defensive or unprofessional. And ethically, we can't disclose our side without violating a patient's privacy.

Most of us aren't here just to "do a job." We want to be excellent. We want to be trusted. We want to be liked. We want people to come back — not because they have to, but because they want to. And most of the time, that's what happens. But not always.

Sometimes you meet someone who doesn't like you no matter what you do. Someone unhappy with their own life. Someone who feels powerful only when tearing others down. That's part of practicing medicine. And honestly? Part of life.

So what do we do with all of this? We build thick skin. But thick skin doesn't mean indifference. It doesn't mean shutting down or pretending words don't matter. It means learning how to separate criticism that helps us grow from noise that only wears us down. It means remembering that one bad review doesn't erase years of trust, hundreds of grateful patients, or the quiet thank-yous that never make it online.

Reputation in medicine is fragile. It can be bruised in seconds, yet it's built over decades. We protect it not by fighting every battle in public, but by showing up day after day with consistency, humility, and care.

Thick skin isn't about being hard. It's about being steady. Because the truth is this: What defines us isn't the one person who tears us down. It's the countless lives we lift up.

We learn to hear hard things without letting them shake our foundation. We learn to carry the weight without letting it crush us. We learn that not everyone will like us, and that doesn't mean we're doing it wrong. You will never please everyone. Someone will always find something wrong with you.

In the blur of modern medicine, it's easy to forget who we are outside the white coat. Yet remembering — that's everything. When the system weighs heavy and expectations rise, we're forced back to a deeper question: Who are we when we're not "Doctor?" No single person — no comment, no review — can take that away.

This is thick skin. And in medicine — especially internal medicine — you need it.

These reflections reach deeper — beyond the grind — into purpose: What sustains us, why we stay, and how we fight for the very soul of medicine.

Knowing Your Worth

I've practiced outpatient internal medicine for over a decade, joining my current group straight out of residency. Since then, I've watched the landscape shift — corporate takeovers, tightening regulations, staffing shortages, and endless debates over salary, documentation, and work-life balance.

Reimbursements have been cut. Morale has taken hits, yet that's not an internal medicine problem — it's a healthcare problem. Across each specialty, we're navigating a system that often feels stacked against us.

We don't need more resignations, we need more resolve — physicians who lead. Who advocate for this field and the people we serve.

Patients want a primary care doctor — someone they know. Someone they trust. Someone who sees the whole picture, not just one part.

That's what drew me in, and it's what keeps me here. I've built a system for myself that works. I care for my patients, review labs, document — and protect time at home by keeping work at work. It's not always easy, but it's intentional.

Are there frustrations? Absolutely. Prior authorizations. Endless charting. Yet those aren't unique to internal medicine. They're systemic, and they shouldn't scare anyone away from this field.

Salary and value come up often — and rightly so. Yet here's the truth: If you don't know your worth, no one else will.

PART IV

Identity in the White Coat

We look beyond the grind to the marrow of medicine: purpose. It's why we stay, what sustains us, and how we fight for the soul of this profession. We cannot mend broken systems if, in the process, we lose the humanity within them.

BEHIND DOCTOR IS A HUMAN BEING trying to reconcile the role they play with the person they are. As we move through life, questions of identity echo through our minds, bouncing like a pinball, scattered and relentless. Am I a doctor? A friend? A colleague? A leader? A husband? A parent? A son?

These questions don't arrive suddenly; they linger. They shape how we see ourselves and how others see us. Every day, we're asked to balance who we truly are with who we're expected to be.

In medicine, that balance is fragile. We carry the weight of responsibility, chasing clarity, meaning, and success. We show up for others — giving pieces of ourselves, trying not to lose who we are in the process. We smile. We stay strong. We solve problems we didn't create. We become the one everyone relies on.

But what's expected of us? Every move is scrutinized by the system, by patients, and, perhaps most harshly, by ourselves. Beneath it all, we're still human. We want to be grounded, present. Yet sometimes, we're just tired.

The truth is simple: Work is work, life is life, and there has to be a line. Not knowing that boundary can break you. At some point, you have to stop and ask: What truly matters to me?

Balance isn't a luxury. It's a necessity — for peace, for presence, for the possibility of joy. If things feel off, pause. Reassess. Fix what's broken. Release what's lost. Set boundaries. Let go of what drains you and invest in what fills you. See life not as something to manage but something to live, because life is shorter than we think. Change it now — not someday. "Someday" isn't promised.

For me, the questions that matter most aren't about productivity or prestige. They're about meaning: What do I have? What do I want? How do I get there? And how do I stay whole along the way?

Medicine teaches us resilience, but it can also erode us if we're not careful. Confidence doesn't arrive overnight; it grows slowly, watered by experience and by self-compassion. Doubt, second-guessing, the feeling of falling short — those are part of the journey too.

So I remind myself: I am more than a profession. I'm a dad, a husband, a son, a brother, a friend, a colleague, a leader — who happens to be a doctor. That truth keeps me grounded. That truth keeps me whole.

Ask yourself again: Who are you?

There's a quiet arrogance that can creep into the exam room — often unintentional, but no less damaging. It's the belief that, because we went to medical school, passed our boards, and earned the white coat, our words carry unquestionable authority. Let's be clear: our words are not the gospel. Medicine is not a religion, and physicians are not gods.

Yet somewhere along the way — through our training, our titles, and the expectations placed on us — we are led to believe we must speak with absolute certainty, that every decision must be firm, every explanation flawless, every recommendation final.

Still, anyone who believes their words are that accurate, that absolute, that untouchable is out of touch with the reality of medicine and the humanity of our patients. What medical school provides is knowledge. What practice provides — through years of showing up, falling short, and learning from the people in front of us — is humility.

The truth is, the longer one practices, the more it becomes clear that being a doctor is not about having the right answers. It's about asking the right questions. It's about listening to someone who's scared, confused, overwhelmed, and finding a way to meet them where they are.

Some patients break down in tears before a word is even spoken. Others walk in angry or defensive, convinced they won't be heard. Some can't read their medication bottles. Others carry binders meticulously filled with lab and specialist notes.

What works isn't always what's printed in the guidelines. What works is understanding a patient's fears, beliefs, background, their "why."

Yes, the training matters. The long nights, the exams, the rigor — it's a critical foundation. Yet being well-educated is only half the job. The other half — the part that truly defines good medicine — is connection. It's the ability to talk to someone like a person, not a problem; to recognize when fear is wearing a mask; to see when someone is nodding but not understanding; to hear the weight in someone's silence.

Medicine is science, but it's also story. Each patient brings a narrative, and effective care begins with listening to it. Modern medicine prioritizes speed and efficiency, but connection? That takes time.

Medicine isn't about making decisions. It's about how we deliver them: tone, timing, trust. It's knowing when to be gentle, when to be clear, and when to sit in the discomfort together.

Some days, we're the ones offering solutions; other days, we're steady hands in a storm. Yet we must never confuse expertise with omniscience. We don't enter exam rooms to dictate; we enter to collaborate. Yes. Sometimes we must be firm — when urgency demands action, when life is at stake. Still, even then, the goal is not control. The goal is guidance, advocacy, support.

The old hierarchy of medicine lingers in too many rooms: doctor on the pedestal, patient on the receiving end. Patients are not blank slates; they are teachers. They bring culture, experience, insight, and often, wisdom earned through lived experience. They challenge assumptions. They ask important questions. They remind us that medicine isn't practiced in a vacuum. That's not a threat to our expertise; that's what makes it real.

The minute a physician believes there's nothing left to learn is the minute they stop being a good doctor. Patients don't demand perfection; they seek partnership. They want to feel heard, understood, respected. They want a doctor who explains, not one who lectures. They want someone who speaks with, not down to them — someone who sees beyond the chart.

They deserve honesty. They deserve space to process, to ask

questions, to say no. And when the medical system has failed them — when they've been ignored, dismissed, or mistreated — they deserve someone who restores that trust. They don't want superiority; they want sincerity.

In each patient interaction, we get to choose the role we play. Are we the expert who speaks in absolutes? Or are we the advocate who asks what matters most to the person in front of us? Some days, we need to persuade. Some days, we need to pause. Yet every day, we have the opportunity to build trust — or to break it.

Patients come to us vulnerable, uncertain, often afraid. They deserve more than a treatment plan. They deserve humanity. We're not here to be right. We're here to be helpful, supportive, real. It's time to shift the posture of medicine to less hierarchy, more humanity, less dictation, more dialogue.

The patients who linger in our memory aren't always the ones with rare conditions or dramatic recoveries; they're the ones who let us in, who trusted us with their truth, who reminded us why we chose this profession in the first place. That trust isn't earned through certainty; it's earned through care. Not outpatient clinical care, but human care, eye contact, compassion, humility, presence.

Our words aren't gospel; they're guidance. And the best medicine happens when we stop talking at patients and start talking with them. For in the end, it's not about being right; it's about being there.

That lesson doesn't just apply in the exam room — it applies to us, too. Physicians are quick to offer compassion to others, but slow to offer it to ourselves. We forget that presence matters more than perfection, even in our own lives.

Knowing Our Worth

We look around and compare ourselves to others, measuring progress by someone else's milestones. We seek validation, reassurance, a reason to believe we're doing okay. Yet the more we chase external affirmation, the more distant our own self-worth becomes.

That quiet uneasiness you feel sometimes — the restlessness, the self-doubt, the desperate search for meaning — it's more common than you think. Most of us go through life carrying it like an invisible weight.

I have come to understand that self-worth is not something you're born with — it's something you must constantly cultivate. And if you're not careful, the pursuit of self-worth can backfire. When it's rooted in fear or insecurity, it can become paralyzing. It can spiral into anxiety, depression, decreased self-confidence — issues that are as real and physical as they are psychological.

The body and mind are deeply interconnected. I've seen this in my own life and in the lives of my patients. Chronic stress, self-doubt, internalized pressure — they don't live in our heads. They show up in our bodies. In fatigue. In tension. In sleepless nights and quiet suffering. And when we stop believing in ourselves, everything else begins to unravel.

That's why confidence matters. And I don't mean loud, boastful, performative confidence. I mean the quiet, grounded kind — the kind that says, "I belong here. I'm capable. I may not be perfect. But I am enough."

Confidence isn't arrogance — it's trust: Trust in your process, in your potential, that you can handle whatever comes your way, even if you don't have all the answers right now. It's about believing not only in who you are, but in who you're becoming.

When I chose a less traditional path through the Caribbean, people questioned it. When I submitted my essays to publications, many didn't respond. Some said it didn't fit their style; others didn't say anything at all.

I've always held onto one belief: No one can define my limitations but me. That conviction has carried me through some of the most uncertain chapters of my life.

When I applied to medical school, the message was clear: I wasn't competitive enough. I heard it in rejection after rejection, in the silences that followed my applications, in the polite dismissals that made it sound final. But "final" is a word I've never accepted easily.

Eventually, one school gave me a chance. And when that door opened, I made sure to walk through it with everything I had. I studied harder. I leaned into the grind. I carried the weight of every "no" I had ever heard and turned it into fuel for the "yes" I had finally been given.

Still none of that stopped me. If anything, it pushed me further. For I've realized that rejection doesn't diminish your value; it redirects your path. When we let go of the need for others to validate us, we begin to build something far more lasting: self-respect. And with self-respect comes clarity — clarity in decisions, in purpose, in goals.

We can't live our lives according to someone else's expectations. That's a recipe for disappointment. Sure, we can use others as role models, as sources of inspiration. We can ask for advice. We can listen. Yet at the end of the day, we have to make decisions that align with our values, our goals, our truth.

Setting your own expectations — ones that are high yet grounded in reality — is one of the most empowering things you can do. Because when you're the one setting the bar, you're also the one in control of how you respond when things don't go as planned.

And they won't always go as planned. You'll fail. You'll fall short. You'll second-guess yourself. That's part of it. Each failure is a building block. Each stumble is a step forward. Fail once? Learn. Fail twice? Learn more. Fail again? You're probably closer than you think.

People often ask me how I stay motivated. The answer is simple: I believe in myself. I don't always have all the answers, and I don't always feel confident, but I show up anyway. I write, even when I wonder if anyone's listening. I lead, even when I feel unsure. I try, even when I carry the truth that I might fail. Because the alternative — doing nothing, playing small, waiting for permission — is no longer acceptable to me.

We each have a unique voice, a unique purpose, a unique contribution to make. Yet if we let fear or doubt silence us, we rob the world of what we have to offer. And we rob ourselves of the fulfillment that comes from doing hard things, from persevering, from growing through adversity.

Negativity and denial used to make me question myself. Now, they drive me. They remind me that success isn't handed out — it's earned. Not by being the loudest or the flashiest, but by being persistent. By being intentional. By staying rooted in who you are, even when the world tries to shake that foundation. Not because of your title, your résumé, or your accolades, but because you are you. You care. You try. You keep going, even when it's hard.

So if no one's told you lately: You are allowed to set high goals. You are allowed to define your own success. You are allowed to bet on yourself, even if others don't — especially if others don't.

Physician as Parent

Being a parent is a life of its own. You're not responsible for just your child's survival; you're responsible for their growth, their well-being, their future. It's a responsibility you take on willingly, one that reshapes you completely. And for those of us in medicine, it doesn't only change who we are at home — it also transforms who we are in the exam room.

I had seen patients break down in front of me. I had held their hands during difficult conversations. I had delivered bad news. I thought I knew what it meant to hold someone's life in your hands. Yet, nothing prepared me for what it feels like when that life is your own child's.

My work life doesn't exist in a vacuum — it bends constantly around the needs of the people waiting for me at home. I try to give my patients my full attention, but I'm always aware of the clock. Of baseball practice. Of bedtime stories. Every decision I make at work is filtered through the lens of my family. What time I arrive. How late I stay. Which tasks I finish now, and which ones I push into the margins of the night. I live in two worlds and am deeply committed to both because medicine demands presence, but so does fatherhood and so does love.

It's not easy. The weight of two worlds can feel crushing at times. But it's also what gives my life shape, meaning, and perspective. At the end of the day, I'm not just a doctor who happens to have a family. I'm a husband and father who happens to practice medicine, and I wouldn't trade that truth for anything.

Being a doctor means shouldering the vulnerability of others.

Being a parent means revealing your own. And that vulnerability has taught me more about medicine than any textbook ever could.

Every new symptom in my children felt like a riddle with high stakes. In those moments, I wasn't a physician — I was a parent, powerless in a way I had never known. When my second child came along, I thought I would be better prepared. I was more seasoned, more relaxed, ready to trust myself. But she was different: a different temperament, a different energy, a different gender.

And suddenly, I wasn't the expert anymore. Parenting stripped away the illusion of control that medicine had given me. It reminded me that presence mattered more than certainty, love more than knowledge. And it's that same truth I now carry into the exam room. Parenthood isn't linear; it's humbling. And that humility follows me to work every single day.

The white coat didn't come with me into the nursery. Medical training didn't soothe the midnight cries or answer the endless "what ifs" running through my head. Experience in the exam room didn't guarantee certainty at home. It was humbling. It was human. And it reminded me that love, not knowledge, is the real guide in parenting.

I remember the fear with my firstborn — trying to decipher cries, fevers, late-night worries that something might be wrong. By the time my third child arrived, I had grown into my role. I felt steadier, more grounded. Even now, I'm constantly learning — from scraped knees to broken hearts, from tantrums to quiet moments of connection. The first words, first steps, first haircut are etched into my memory in a way no medical achievement ever could be. Mood, behavior, emotions — each new stage feels like uncharted territory. Just when I think I've figured out the playbook, my children rewrite it. They teach me something new.

Parenting demands constant adjustment. There's no fixed formula, no textbook to consult, no algorithm to follow. And yet, in that chaos, there is magic. Watching them reach milestones, discover confidence, and grow into themselves is one of the most rewarding experiences of my life. It reminds me that the most profound lessons don't always come from medicine. Sometimes, they come from bedtime stories, scraped knees, or the quiet courage of a child learning to stand on their own.

They've taught me how to be more patient, how to manage my emotions, how to recalibrate my priorities. They've shaped me into a better leader, a better mentor — someone worth looking up to. I carry that responsibility with me always. I never want to be anything less than my best for them. That's a standard I've set for myself, and one I'll never stop striving to meet.

I learn something new every day, every minute, every second. There's never a moment when I'm not learning from my kids. And that standard spills over into medicine.

When I care for my patients — especially young adults or elderly parents — I don't just see a diagnosis. I see someone's child. Someone's mother. Someone's father. I see their fears reflected in my own. I hear echoes of my own anxieties in their questions. And more often than not, I picture my own kids and ask myself: How would I want their doctor to treat them? That question guides me more than any protocol. It softens my tone, lengthens my patience, and reminds me that compassion must be as deliberate as any prescription.

When I'm at work, I give my patients everything I have. But even in the middle of a busy day, part of me wonders what I'm missing at home. The bedtime stories I didn't read. The math homework I didn't help with. The scraped knee I wasn't there to clean.

That guilt can be heavy, but I've come to see it differently. The weight of that tension is proof that I care deeply about both parts of my life. It's not a failing. It's a reminder of my humanity.

I'll never get it perfectly right. No one does. But the very fact that I wrestle with the balance tells me something important: that both medicine and family matter too much for me not to feel pulled between them. And maybe that's the truest measure of love: caring enough to feel the strain.

Parenthood. Medicine. Sometimes, the lines between them blur. I've had patients ask me about parenting — how to manage tantrums, how to cope with a teenager's anxiety, how to juggle their careers with family life. I don't answer as a physician; I answer as a fellow parent. I share what's worked in my own home, what hasn't, and the reminder that none of us is doing it "right" — we're all just trying our best.

Those conversations are never billed or charted. But they're some of the most meaningful I have because they remind me that medicine is not only about treatment — it's about connection. How to be present, even in a world that demands constant motion — that's what my children have taught me. They've softened me. Grounded me. Given me a reason to put the pager down and walk out of the office when the workday ends. And in a profession that can so easily pull you into burnout and bureaucracy, that reminder — that grounding — is everything.

They've taught me how to listen, how to slow down, how to notice the small things.

Parenting hasn't distracted me from being a better doctor; it's the reason I've become one.

Walking a Tightrope

Life doesn't hand out balance — it demands it. Some days I feel like walking a tightrope: arms outstretched, suspended in midair, the world below watching every move. Sometimes there's a harness; sometimes not. Sometimes there's a bar to help center me. It feels like comfort — but is it an illusion?

That's the paradox of balance: You don't know if the safety net is there until you fall.

So how do you approach a moment like that? Do you step out expecting the worst? Or do you trust the practice, the preparation, the countless small lessons that brought you here and take the step anyway?

Preparation is everything. Complacency is what causes the fall. The more you work on your craft, on yourself, the steadier your footing becomes. Even then, the pressure never fully lets up.

We've all been on that tightrope: trying to please everyone, trying not to let anyone down, trying to keep it all together, wanting to succeed while quietly unraveling, wanting to be enough for your family, your team, your profession, for yourself. It's a roller coaster that never stops, and the question becomes: How do we balance it all without losing ourselves? As a physician, I've been there. I've lived all of it.

This is a demanding field. At best, perfection is the standard — at worst, even perfection falls short. You're expected to meet everyone's expectations; to never make a mistake; to be happy, composed, and available no matter what's happening inside; to lead by example; to mentor those around you; you offer uplifting guidance when you're running on empty; to be a shoulder to cry on, even when your own shoulders are burdened.

These aren't theoretical expectations; they're the unspoken rules of the profession, and they take a toll. In medicine, we're asked to give so much of ourselves that sometimes we forget there's a self to protect. The pressure isn't a wave; it's constant, quiet, unrelenting. And still, we show up. We walk that tightrope day after day.

No one sees the tremble in your hands. No one hears the doubt in your head. For in our world — whether it's medicine, leadership, or business — any sign of struggle can be mistaken for weakness, and weakness can shake your reputation, your confidence, your identity.

The truth is that this isn't about medicine. This is about being human in a world that doesn't always allow space for humanity. We are terrified of failure, but failure is not the enemy. In truth, you only fail if you try, and you only grow if you try. You can only overcome failure if you acknowledge it.

I've failed, as have the most successful people you know. What separates those who grow from those who don't isn't perfection — it's persistence. It's the choice to keep moving forward, to take the next step, to walk anyway.

There is no finish line for perfection. The closer you get, the further it moves. Solve one issue, and another takes its place. Meet one goal, and a new one appears.

Life doesn't pause for us to catch up; it keeps moving — faster than we expect, indifferent to our pace. Chasing perfection is like running after a horizon: No matter how far you go, it never gets closer. What matters isn't reaching it, it's learning to live, grow, and find meaning along the way.

So how do we cope? How do we deal with the numbness, the insecurity, the exhaustion of trying to do everything for everyone?

Choose to seek joy — not as a reward, but as a necessity. Protect the people closest to you. Carve out time for what truly matters. Because when you do, you rediscover something essential: perspective.

Remember that life is bigger than your titles. Bigger than your roles. Bigger than what others expect of you. Along the way, you'll meet all kinds of people — some who support you, some who challenge you, and some who simply don't understand you. That's part of the process. Those are the growing pains of becoming, of learning when to push forward, when to hold steady, and when to let go.

We can't control every twist in the rope, but we can control how we walk. We can prepare for unpredictability. We can anticipate struggle. We can expect to stumble — but we don't have to fall apart. And when it feels like too much — when the rope sways and the pressure builds — sometimes the strongest thing you can do is pause and recenter.

Here's the truth about that tightrope: It's only as narrow as you believe it to be. If you see it as fear, it becomes fear. If you see it as a challenge, you rise. The rope is nothing more than an imaginary line.

The reason others seem to walk it with ease — doing flips, dives, and impossible maneuvers — isn't because they're fearless. It's because they've stopped shrinking themselves to fit the rope. They've expanded their perspective until the rope feels like a path. They don't walk differently; they see differently. And that changes everything.

Peace is not the prize for the perfect; it's the mindset of those who keep going. It's not tied to a paycheck, or a title, or applause.

Just when you think you've found your footing, comparison sneaks in. But comparison doesn't have to bring you down. It can be a reminder that your path is your own, that worth isn't measured side-by-side, that balance looks different for everyone. Balance is not tied to titles, or paychecks, or applause. It's tied to perspective, to presence, to purpose.

So if you're out there — arms outstretched, walking that rope — know this: You don't have to be flawless. You don't have to have it all figured out. You just have to keep going — not for them, not for the title, not for the illusion of control, but because persistence itself is proof you're still becoming.

Casting a Critical Eye

Everything people do, say, or post seems to invite scrutiny. I can't pinpoint exactly when that shift happened, but I suspect the pandemic years played a role. During COVID, we were isolated, anxious, and glued to our screens. Every decision — to mask, to gather, to vaccinate — became fodder for endless debate. And the hypercritical spirit that took root during those months didn't vanish when the world reopened. It lingered. It stuck with us. And in many ways, it still shapes the way we see one another.

It feels like the world has become more critical. Not in the sense of asking questions or offering constructive feedback, but in a way that borders on relentless judgment. And I feel it too. I catch myself setting impossible standards — expecting flawless performance, perfect choices, unshakable calm. But what does that serve? The more I look at it, the more I realize: It serves no one.

Constant criticism doesn't inspire growth; it fuels anxiety, breeds resentment, feeds the gnawing sense of never being enough. And if that's the standard we hold ourselves to, we'll never learn to extend grace to others or to ourselves.

I see this pattern most clearly in medicine.

As physicians, we're trained to be critical thinkers — to analyze symptoms, sift through lab results, weigh risks against benefits. The who, what, where, when, why, and how are drilled into us from day one. And in that context, critical thinking is vital; a missed detail can mean the difference between life and death.

But somewhere along the way, that critical eye we're trained to use outwardly turns inward. What starts as vigilance can harden into perfectionism. What begins as discipline can blur into self-judgment. We magnify flaws. We hold colleagues, patients, and ourselves to standards that are often unrealistic. I've seen simple conversations — ones that should have been moments of reassurance — turn into interrogations, as though the goal were to expose weakness rather than foster understanding.

Still, somewhere along the way, that professional vigilance can spill over into how we view ourselves and others outside the exam room. We become hyper-aware of mistakes. This constant state of criticism isn't sustainable. It erodes trust in teams, it dampens morale, and it creates an atmosphere where no one feels safe to be human.

Feedback, when offered with respect and purpose, can sharpen skills and push us forward. I think back to my medical training, when attendings would question me in front of a team. At the time, the barrage of questions felt brutal. Yet looking back, many of those moments were rooted in a desire to teach, to prepare me for the demands of real-world medicine.

There is, of course, a time and place to be critical. Constructive criticism is how we learn. The difference was intention. Those critiques were aimed at growth, not at tearing me down. They were specific, timely, and ultimately useful.

What I worry about now is that we've blurred that line. Criticism has become reflexive rather than purposeful. Instead of being a tool for improvement, it's often an outlet for frustration or an attempt to assert control. That kind of criticism benefits no one. It chips away at self-worth, it creates unnecessary conflict, and it replaces curiosity with judgment.

I don't think this culture of criticism is limited to medicine — it's everywhere. Scroll through social media for five minutes and you'll see it: every post dissected, every opinion challenged, every mistake amplified. The court of public opinion rarely shows mercy. And while some accountability can be healthy, more often it feels like piling on for sport.

It's a cycle that breeds more fear than growth, more noise than clarity. And it's exhausting. The cost is subtle but profound. We start to second-guess ourselves. We hesitate to take risks or to speak up. Creativity shrinks. Anxiety grows. The constant expectation of being critiqued — by others or by ourselves — becomes a weight we carry everywhere.

And in medicine, that weight is heavy enough already. Doctors live under the pressure of perfection, often imposed by systems that expect flawless performance without acknowledging human limits. When we add relentless self-criticism and peer criticism to the mix, burnout becomes almost inevitable.

So what's the alternative? I think it begins with patience — with others, but perhaps more importantly, with ourselves. Patience doesn't mean lowering standards. It doesn't mean ignoring mistakes or letting go of accountability. It means accepting that people are human, that growth takes time, and that empathy often accomplishes more than judgment ever could.

When I lead with patience — asking what got in the way, listening without judgment — I almost always learn more. Maybe the problem was the cost of medication. Maybe it was the fatigue of juggling two jobs. Maybe it was fear. When I step back from criticism, I create space for connection. And in medicine, that connection is often the most healing thing we have to offer.

In leadership, I've learned that criticism alone doesn't motivate anyone. It may correct a behavior, but more often it discourages the person behind it. Far more effective is to listen, to encourage, to correct gently but clearly. People rise when they feel supported, not when they feel scrutinized.

Of course, none of this works if we can't first quiet the critic within ourselves. Most of us carry an inner voice that nitpicks every decision, every action, every word.

Mine can be relentless. It tells me I should have said more in that meeting, that I should have written a stronger essay, that I should have been more patient with my kids at the end of a long day. That voice never disappears completely, but I'm learning not to let it define me.

Over time, I've come to see that the voice will always be there. I'm learning to treat it less like a judge and more like a reminder. Instead of letting it paralyze me, I pause and ask: Is this criticism useful, or is it just noise? If it's useful, I act on it. If it's noise, I let it go. That shift doesn't silence the critic, but it keeps me moving forward. And maybe that's the real lesson: Growth isn't about eliminating doubt, but about learning how to walk with it.

The world doesn't need more critics. It needs more people willing to understand. To approach situations with calm, with respect, with empathy. Most of us are doing the best we can with the circumstances we're given. Life is complicated. Medicine is complicated. Relationships are complicated. What looks like failure on the surface often has a story underneath it.

We don't need to abandon criticism altogether. But we need to restore it to its proper place: as a tool for growth, not as a default mode of interaction. When we make that shift, we create space for patience, for kindness, and for trust.

And maybe that's the most important lesson. Criticism may sharpen skills, but compassion sustains people. Without the latter, the former loses its power. "I want more patients."

"I want fewer call shifts."

"I want a better office."

"I want to make more money."

So often, those wants aren't rooted in purpose; they're rooted in perception. We assume others have it better, that their lives are easier, more fulfilling. And that's where the trap begins.

Comparison rarely tells us the full story. It feeds the illusion that someone else's highlight reel is reality — while our own struggles are proof of inadequacy. We chase someone else's life without fully knowing what that life even is. We romanticize the unknown and lose sight of what's already good. The grass isn't greener — it's different, and sometimes, it's not even real.

I remember being a med student, desperate to get out of basic sciences. I couldn't wait to start rotations. When I finally did, I wanted to be in residency. And once residency started, all I could think about was getting into practice.

I was always comparing myself to those ahead of me — always looking up the ladder, wondering when I'd finally feel like I had arrived. It stole my joy. It dulled my motivation. It made me feel stuck — like I was always behind, always falling short.

I spent years measuring myself against people who had already finished what I was struggling to survive. And all it gave me was anxiety — anxiety that I'd fail, that I wasn't good enough, that I wasn't becoming the kind of doctor I was "supposed" to be. Comparison didn't make me better; it made me scared.

But you define your success. You own who you are and who you're becoming. When you compare yourself to mentors, colleagues, or role models, it's not about envy — it's about aspiration. It can show you what's possible. It can push you forward, not hold you back.

The danger isn't in comparing — it's in comparing blindly to people you don't know, to lives you don't understand, to curated highlight reels that skip the struggle.

Don't measure yourself against a version of success that isn't real. Instead, compare yourself to who you were yesterday, and to people whose lives reflect the one you truly want — not just the one that photographs well. Fix what's draining your energy. Stop the irrational measuring. And when comparison sneaks in, own who you are and what you bring to the table.

And as for your weaknesses? That's where growth lives. Acknowledge what you lack and build on it, because what feels like a weakness today can become tomorrow's strength. And when that happens, you won't need to compare anymore. You'll have become the person you used to envy.

Here's the irony: The person we underestimate most is usually ourselves. To our patients, however, we are more than enough.

So stop measuring your worth by someone else's wins and start defining success on your terms. Joy isn't found in chasing someone else's story, it's found in owning your own.

Pausing for Celebration

We work so hard to achieve, and then when we do, what happens? We move on. Quickly. Quietly. As if the victory was expected, inevitable, or somehow not worthy of a moment's reflection. We barely acknowledge it. We look toward the next goal, the next deadline, the next thing on the horizon.

You deserve to celebrate your successes. You deserve to feel the joy, the relief, and the pride that comes with accomplishing something meaningful. These moments are not stepping stones — they're the culmination of your effort, resilience, and growth, and they should be honored as such.

I'll be the first to admit: I've struggled with this. For years, I lived in the mindset of "what's next?" Medical school? Done. Residency? Check. Build a practice? Achieved. Raise a family? Ongoing. Each time I reached a goal, I created another. Every milestone was met with more pressure, more urgency, more expectations — mostly from myself.

The problem with that approach is that it creates an endless loop. You never feel done. You never feel like it's enough. As soon as you arrive at one destination, you're already packing for the next journey. The danger of this mindset isn't burnout — it's disconnection. You lose touch with the "why" behind it all. You forget to notice how far you've come.

It's like worry. You stress about something until that issue is resolved — then your brain finds a new problem. It's a form of survival mode, constantly scanning for threats or unmet expectations. And while that can drive achievement, it also robs you of peace.

So here's the shift I've tried to make and encourage you to make too: Stop and look back — not to dwell, but to appreciate. Reflect on how far you've come. Think about the version of yourself who once wished for what you have now. Let that be a source of motivation, but also of grounding.

There's power in that pause.

The countless hours of studying, doubting, and pushing through.

The sacrifices made in silence.

The moments of uncertainty you faced but kept going anyway.

The people you supported and the ones who supported you.

The small wins that piled up into something bigger.

The version of yourself that kept showing up — even when it was hard.

Those things matter. They deserve acknowledgment and not once, but often.

I think about the years of training. The uncertainty I carried during residency, the way I grew into my role as a physician, husband, and father. The time I questioned my ability, my worth, my path — and found my way through. When I do that, I'm reminded not of the struggle, but of the growth. It's like seeing your own life with new eyes.

One of the ways I stay connected to this perspective is by checking in with myself regularly. I revisit my own story — intentionally. That reflection becomes fuel. It's a guide for future growth, yes, but it's also a reminder of resilience, of purpose, of how capable we are when we don't give up.

None of this means you should stop setting goals. Quite the opposite. Growth is essential and progress is fulfilling. It should be paired with appreciation. You can move forward while honoring the ground you've already covered.

Just as we should celebrate success, we should also value failure — it teaches us how to grow better and wiser.

Failure is not the opposite of success; it's part of the path, a detour that often holds more insight than a straight road. When things don't go as planned, when you fall short or face a setback, ask yourself:

What did I learn?

What could I do differently?

How can I turn this into something useful?

Some of the most important truths in my life have come from moments that felt like failure: Not matching at a dream program, receiving tough feedback, struggling through moments of burnout, rejections of my writing. These were not easy seasons, but they were shaping ones. They taught me more about who I am — and who I want to become — than any accolade ever could.

When we use failure as feedback, we become more well-rounded. We grow thicker skin, sharper minds, and softer hearts. We learn humility. We learn strategy. We learn empathy for ourselves and for others walking their own rocky paths.

So wherever you are in your journey — whether you're on a high or in a valley — pause. Take a deep breath. Look back with honesty and look ahead with hope. Acknowledge what you've achieved. Let it strengthen you. Let it inspire you. And when you fall short, as we all do, don't run from it. Sit with it. Ask what it's trying to teach you. Use it, then move forward — with more clarity, more grace, and more resilience.

Success is a moment. Failure is a moment. Your story is what ties them together. Make it a story you're proud to tell.

Anticipation and Speculation

I've spent years second-guessing myself — wondering what others thought, how I measured up, whether I was doing enough. The older I get, the more I realize something simple and true: Overthinking robs the present of its meaning and replaces it with ghosts of what if. It drags us into imaginary futures, each one more anxiety-ridden than the last. It disguises itself as preparation, but it's really just worry in a lab coat.

What if this visit goes badly? What if the doctor is late? What if the labs are abnormal? What if it's something serious? What if the treatment doesn't work?

Of course, sometimes speculation bends toward hope: Maybe I'll get good news today, maybe this medicine will finally help. Yet more often, it breeds anxiety. And even when our guesses are right, we've already paid the toll by living through it twice: once in our minds and again in real time. And the truth is, our speculation is usually wrong.

I see it in my office every day. A patient walks in visibly nervous. They've spent days googling, spiraling, imagining the worst. By the end of the visit, their shoulders relax. The diagnosis wasn't what they feared. The plan is manageable. The reality was far more grounded than the monster they built in their heads.

They often say, "I wish I hadn't spent so much time worrying." I wish they hadn't, too. Still, I understand it. We speculate because we want control. We try to predict outcomes so we can prepare ourselves, shield ourselves. It's a defense mechanism. It's also a trap, because speculation isn't clarity; it's clutter and it disconnects us from what's happening.

There's a big difference between anticipation and speculation, and I try to teach this to my patients and to myself.

Anticipation is grounded in fact. I'm going on vacation next week. I'm looking forward to it. That's anticipation. There's no guessing, no spiraling — it's rooted in something real. Speculation, on the other hand, is different. What if the flight gets delayed? What if I get sick? What if it rains the whole time? And suddenly, what should have been joyful is drowned in anxiety about things that haven't even happened — and probably never will.

I see the same dynamic with new medications. A patient gets a prescription and immediately starts speculating: What if I get side effects? What if it doesn't work? What if it makes me worse? They haven't taken a single pill, yet they've already imagined three bad outcomes.

And I get it: Caution is human. But speculation often leads to resistance, nonadherence, and unnecessary stress. Speculation keeps us from living in the truth of the moment. It replaces facts with fear. Instead of asking, "what's true right now?" we drift into "what if everything goes wrong later?" And when we do that, we don't just rob ourselves of peace, we rob ourselves of joy.

Joy can't coexist with mental chaos. It lives in clarity, in presence, in simplicity.

As a doctor, I've had to learn this lesson the hard way. I've speculated about patients before — worried about outcomes, imagined complications, stressed over what could happen. All it does is steal time and mental space I could've used to be fully present for them and for myself. And in my personal life, as a parent, a husband, a leader, speculation has creeped in: Am I doing enough? Did I disappoint someone? Can I keep all the pieces together?

Those thoughts rarely lead to action; they lead to doubt. Here's the truth: We can't prevent the unknown, we can't predict every outcome, yet we can choose not to live inside our fears before they become real. We can meet each moment as it comes: with curiosity instead of control. We're allowed to not know yet and we're allowed to wait.

So if you're reading this and you're caught in your own spiral of what-ifs about your health, your future, your career, your relationships, let me offer this: Speculation may feel like preparation, but more often than not, it's a thief in disguise. Come back to what you know. Come back to what's real. Joy lives there, and you deserve to feel it, without apology.

Be an Inspiration

You must inspire yourself before you can inspire others. Believe in your craft. Believe in what you do. Believe in you. That belief echoes through everything you touch. It transforms struggle into strength, and doubt into direction. Inner peace creates outer peace. Inner happiness becomes shared happiness. It starts within, and it spreads everywhere.

Patients look up to us — not only as physicians, but as people. Some of mine come in dressed like they're headed to a ball. Hair done. Lipstick perfect. Outfit immaculate. Maybe they're not dressing up for me; maybe they're doing it for them because for them, this moment, this visit, matters. They don't ask about blood pressure or medications. They ask about life. They want to know how to feel better, live better, be better. How do I manage to work out, raise a family, and show up for them while also not losing myself?

They're not listening for advice; they're looking for inspiration. And although I don't feel extraordinary, I show up, I make space. I let my life speak louder than my credentials.

Being an inspiration isn't about prestige or titles. It's a privilege, a responsibility, an opportunity to change lives — not only with medicine, but with presence, with the act of being wholly there.

Every day, I try. I talk with my patients, not at them. I meet them on common ground. I don't stand above them, I stand beside them. And for many, that alone feels rare: to have a doctor who listens, who sees, who relates. I hold myself to a standard not just to treat, but to inspire. And here's the quiet truth I've learned: The more I inspire them, the more they inspire me. It's a loop. What you give off is what others receive. And when they carry it forward — to their families, their communities, their own lives — it multiplies. It circulates. It outlives the exam room.

Inspiration isn't a title. It's not an award, or a nameplate on a door. It's a feeling, an energy. It's the quiet knowing that who you are or something you did made a difference.

I love what I do. I'm passionate about it. And that passion deepens every time I see a patient smile, every time they reach a goal, every time they feel proud of themselves — because I'm proud of them, too. That's the heartbeat of this work: Not just healing, but uplifting; not just treating, but empowering; not just prescribing, but partnering.

On Love and Partnerships

People say marriage is hard. People say medicine is hard. I chose both. Over time, I came to see that medicine and marriage don't simply coexist — they collide. At times, they crash into each other with the full weight of stress, time constraints, emotional exhaustion, and the sheer complexity of trying to care deeply for others both inside and outside your home. Medicine demands a lot; marriage deserves even more. The missed dinners, the emotional fatigue. They don't measure the constant tension between duty and presence, the silent weight so many physicians carry home at night. The pressure is real, and over time, it adds up.

Life felt simpler back then. We were two college kids splitting late-night pizzas, trading dreams about futures still too hazy to name. We didn't know the full road ahead — the long hours, the time apart, the weight of responsibility — but we never doubted our ability to endure it together. Each challenge became another reason to lean in, to trust, to keep going. And with every step, we proved what we had always believed: Whatever waited on the road, we would walk it side by side.

I met Farah in college, before I even knew for sure that I wanted to go to medical school, before the MCAT, before applications, before the grind. Many relationships don't survive long distance. It takes commitment, sacrifice, and an almost stubborn devotion. We had to believe that the temporary hardship was in service of something bigger, something lasting.

When I decided to pursue medicine, everything changed. I left the country to attend medical school abroad, and suddenly we weren't just growing as individuals — we were growing apart in miles, in time zones, in daily routines.

We adapted the best we could. She flew down when she could; I came home when I had breaks. We talked as often as possible. Sometimes it was rushed and tired, squeezed between study sessions and sleep. Sometimes it was filled with frustration. But it was always honest. We didn't pretend it was easy. We were learning how to be apart while holding onto us.

Looking back, I realize how profoundly medicine shaped not just my career, but our relationship. The journey from college to medical school, to residency, to life as a full-time attending — that wasn't my path. It was ours. We both sacrificed. We both matured. We both had to learn how to support each other while also discovering ourselves. And we had to do all of that under the strain of an often-relentless profession.

Being a doctor means wearing many emotional hats. You toggle between outpatient clinical detachment and deep compassion multiple times a day. You hold the pain of strangers and try not to bring it home. But, of course you do. You're human, and when you walk in the door at the end of a long day, there's no magic switch that turns off the physician and turns on the spouse.

Sometimes, after 12 hours of listening, explaining, and absorbing other people's fears, you come home depleted — not because you don't love the person waiting for you, but because there's nothing left to give that day. And that's hard. It's hard for you, and it's even harder for them.

That's the hardest part of dual identity: being a doctor and a partner. These roles require different skills, different energy, different emotional bandwidths. And sometimes they compete with each other.

Over time, we've learned how to navigate that space. We've learned what to share and what to hold. Some stories from work are too heavy, too sacred, or too complex. Other stories are worth sharing, because they let our worlds overlap. And sometimes, we don't need words at all — we need understanding.

One of the most important truths I have come to understand is that presence matters more than perfection. I may not always be home on time. I may carry stress on my shoulders even after I walk through the door. If I can show up honestly — if I can be present, listen, and remain open — then we can keep growing together.

That's life, yet when you go through it all together, year after year, those challenges don't stack up, they shape you. With every new obstacle, more layers of each person are revealed. You grow not as individuals, but as a unit. And with every hardship you overcome, the bond deepens. That's what makes a relationship stronger — not avoiding struggle, but enduring it side by side.

We've faced multiple tests along the way, moments that could have broken us, but instead built us. We've encountered roadblocks, detours, and unexpected speed bumps.

Marriage is a partnership, but it's also a practice, just like medicine. You show up. You work at it. You learn from your mistakes. You try to be better tomorrow than you were yesterday. And you don't do it alone. That's the beauty of it: Neither medicine nor marriage is meant to be a solo endeavor.

But marriage demanded something different. The guilt crept in. Was I a good enough partner? Was I too emotionally closed off? Was I present enough for the people I love? That tension never fully disappears. Over the years, we stopped searching for perfect balance and started striving instead for rhythm.

Some seasons tested us more than others. Residency was brutal: odd hours, chronic fatigue, emotional whiplash. And still, we found moments of connection. We celebrated small wins. We leaned into grace. Because love, like medicine, requires forgiveness. It requires the courage to grow beside someone whose life is constantly being reshaped by a calling.

Now, as a full-time attending and department chair, I see our life as one built not in spite of the challenges, but because of them. We are stronger because we endured. We learned that "hard" doesn't mean something is wrong; it means we're human, and we're doing something that matters.

Being married to a doctor isn't easy. Being married while being a doctor is a different kind of challenge. It means acknowledging when you're stretched too thin. It means checking in. It means listening even when you're tired. It means showing up even when you feel like you have nothing left. Above all, it means choosing each other again and again, no matter how chaotic the day.

Farah knew me before I was "Doctor." She knew me when I was Ryan, a college kid with a big dream and a long way to go. Somehow, she stayed beside me as that dream took shape. She stayed through the all-nighters, the absences, the uncertainties. She stayed through the highs and the heartbreaks.

And I stayed too. Not just for medicine, but for her. At the end of the day, my career gives me purpose, but my marriage gives me meaning.

We're never perfect, but always human. We have hard days, yet we've built a life where medicine and marriage don't have to compete. They can coexist. They can even complement one another — with patience, with practice, and with the deep belief that love isn't about avoiding the storm, but about learning to dance in the rain.

Entering a New World

That lesson — patience, persistence, and the willingness to grow through discomfort — followed me beyond the walls of marriage and medicine. I didn't realize how deeply I had internalized it until years later, when I began writing in earnest and eventually set out to bring a manuscript into the world.

Writing started quietly. It wasn't originally a career goal or even a structured ambition. It was simply a place where thoughts that felt too heavy or complex to carry alone could live safely outside of me. After long days in clinic, I found myself returning to the keyboard, trying to make sense of moments that stayed with me long after patients left the exam room. Writing became less about storytelling and more about understanding — understanding medicine, understanding patients, and in many ways, understanding myself.

I remember one evening sitting alone in my office long after the clinic lights had dimmed. The cleaning crew had already passed through the hallway. The glow of my computer screen reflected off stacks of patient charts and unfinished notes scattered across my desk. I stared at a completed manuscript draft, the cursor blinking at the bottom of the final page, unsure whether to feel relief or vulnerability. Hitting "send" on that first submission felt strangely similar to placing a diagnosis in a patient's chart — an act that carries certainty outward while quietly holding uncertainty underneath. I hesitated longer than I expected before finally pressing the button, realizing in that moment that the manuscript no longer belonged entirely to me.

Completing that manuscript was one of the most demanding creative challenges I had ever faced. It required months — eventually years — of reflection, revision, and emotional honesty. Finishing that final sentence felt monumental. There is something deeply satisfying about seeing a completed manuscript exist as a tangible reflection of countless early mornings, late nights, and quiet moments of doubt.

But I quickly learned that finishing a manuscript is not the culmination of writing. It is the beginning of publishing.

Publishing introduced me to a completely different type of endurance. Writing asks for creativity and vulnerability. Publishing asks for patience and humility. It requires you to release something deeply personal into a process largely outside your control. Developmental editing reshapes structure. Line editing refines voice. Formatting, cover design, marketing, and distribution add layers of complexity that most readers never see. Each stage strengthens the work, but each also demands time and trust.

Medicine had trained me to act decisively. In clinical practice, time carries urgency. When abnormal results return, decisions follow quickly. Patients depend on clarity, even when certainty is impossible. Publishing operates under a different rhythm. Submissions are reviewed slowly. Proposals sit unanswered. Responses, when they come, often arrive weeks or months after emotional investment has already taken root.

That waiting forced me to confront a discomfort I had spent most of my life avoiding: the inability to control outcomes through effort alone.

I learned to tolerate rejection more easily than silence. Rejection, at least, provides resolution. Silence invites uncertainty — the lingering question of whether your work has been read, dismissed, or simply lost among countless other voices hoping to be heard. That uncertainty pushed me to reflect on my motivation for writing in the first place.

At the beginning, I was searching for validation. I wanted reassurance that the experiences shaping my understanding of medicine mattered beyond my own perspective. Seeing my name attached to a published essay felt like confirmation that my reflections held value outside the confines of my own thoughts.

Over time, that motivation shifted. Recognition became less important than resonance. I stopped asking whether my words were being noticed and began asking whether they were connecting. I wanted my writing to reach physicians navigating the same internal conflicts I often felt but rarely voiced. I wanted patients to see the human complexity that exists behind clinical decisions. Writing transformed from personal expression into shared conversation.

As I explored ways to bring a full manuscript to readers, I encountered the realities of the publishing landscape. Self-publishing offered independence and creative control but demanded complete responsibility for editing, distribution, and visibility. Hybrid publishing provided professional guidance but often required significant financial investment. Traditional publishing carried broader reach and institutional credibility but required navigating literary agents, proposals, and prolonged uncertainty.

Each path presented opportunities. Each required compromise. More importantly, each reinforced a lesson I had been learning across multiple chapters of my life: meaningful pursuits rarely unfold according to personal timelines.

Despite the logistical complexities, writing remained deeply personal. I am a physician who writes, not a writer trying to become a physician. Writing is not how I earn my living. It is how I process it. It allows me to reflect on the emotional weight of medicine, the responsibility of leadership, and the evolving understanding of identity that comes with caring for others. My goal has never been literary prestige or financial reward. My goal has always been connection — the possibility that someone reading my words might feel less isolated in their own experiences.

What I did not anticipate was how profoundly writing would reshape my perspective on relationships and personal growth.

Writing expanded my world in subtle but meaningful ways. It introduced me to communities of readers and colleagues who viewed medicine through lenses I had never considered. It also gave me language to better understand relationships that had already begun shaping my life long before I ever placed words on a page.

One of those relationships was with Farah.

I met Farah years earlier, before medical school, during a time when I was still trying to understand who I was becoming. Writing did not lead me to Farah. She had already been part of my life long before I ever began writing.

Meeting her marked the beginning of a chapter defined by partnership, shared growth, and the realization that some of life's most meaningful transitions unfold gradually rather than through dramatic turning points.

She entered my life at a time when I had begun to better understand who I was professionally and creatively, but I was still learning who I was personally. Our relationship deepened my appreciation for balance, emotional presence, and the importance of building a life that extended beyond career milestones and personal ambition.

Looking back, it is striking how closely writing and relationships mirror one another. Both require patience. Both demand honesty. Both evolve through revision, compromise, and trust. Neither follows a predictable timeline, and neither succeeds without vulnerability.

Writing helped me find my voice. Farah helped me understand how to share that voice within a partnership built on mutual respect and shared growth.

Together, those experiences reshaped my understanding of fulfillment. Success was no longer defined solely by professional achievement or creative output. It became defined by connection

— connection to patients, to readers, and ultimately, to the person who would share my life outside the walls of medicine.

The Value of Being Persistent

In medicine, I learned that persistence saves lives. In writing, persistence carries words into the world. Publishing is hard. It's slow. It's unpredictable. Yet it's also worth it for the simple reason that words matter.

I'm in it to spread the word. What began as doubt becomes conviction. What endures is not certainty, but compassion, persistence, and the courage to keep showing up — whether in the exam room or on the page.

That same persistence has shaped every part of my life, including the most important relationship I've ever had. I didn't meet Farah in a lecture hall or at a party. It started with something much simpler: a Facebook message. On my birthday, a stranger wished me well. We shared the same birthday, though I didn't know her, or her brother she mentioned in passing. At the time, it felt like nothing more than a small, random gesture. Looking back now, it was the beginning of something spectacular.

From that message came a conversation. From that conversation, a meeting. From that meeting, a connection we never let go. College was simple in hindsight. We were both just trying to get by — passing classes, figuring out what came next. Our biggest worries were exams and weekends. Neither of us knew where life would lead.

Never did I imagine I'd end up in medical school — let alone in a foreign country. And she certainly didn't picture herself supporting a partner walking such a winding road. While I was navigating classes and clinics abroad, she was finishing college back home. It was hard, lonely, stretching us thin, filled with uncertainty. But we supported each other. We sacrificed. We changed. We grew. And somehow, we overcame it together.

Now here we are, living a life we never could have imagined back then. Still side by side. She is my biggest supporter, my voice of reason, the one who calls me out when I'm wrong and reminds me when I'm right. She prays for me on the hardest days, and I'm endlessly grateful for her faith, her steadiness, her love.

Because the truth is, this doesn't happen by accident. You need someone who sees your goals as clearly as their own. Who believes in you when you're uncertain. Who lifts you higher but also keeps you grounded. That's not just a spouse. That's a best friend, a teammate, a true partner in every sense of the word.

What we've built didn't come from chance. It came from passion, from determination, from two people who refused to give up on each other. What started with a simple birthday message became a life anchored in sacrifice, support, and shared vision. Through uncertainty, distance, and doubt we kept showing up.

That's the lesson: When two people both want it — when they're patient, persistent, and willing to fight for one another — it works. It takes effort. It takes sacrifice. It takes choosing each other, again and again.

That partnership — the rhythm of supporting and being supported — is the same rhythm that carries me through medicine. Farah's belief in me makes me a better doctor. Her honesty keeps me grounded. Her patience reminds me to slow down and listen.

Medicine may be central to my life, but love is what makes it sustainable. And just as I've learned in marriage, the truth in medicine is the same: It isn't about staying — it's about building. Brick by brick, choice by choice, day after day.

Lessons from My Dad

Any time I drifted into envy or entitlement, my parents were quick to ground me. They weren't harsh, but they were clear: Be grateful. Work hard. Stay humble.

My dad modeled that better than anyone. He was a physician, and though he provided well for our family, what stood out wasn't the success — it was the passion. He loved medicine. Not the status, not the title, but the work itself: the problem-solving, the relationships, the privilege of helping people in their most vulnerable moments.

His journey into medicine wasn't easy. He began medical school in Mexico because, even then, getting into a U.S. program was fiercely competitive. Those years were grueling, but he didn't give up. He worked relentlessly, transferred to a U.S. medical school, proved himself, and earned a GI fellowship. His path wasn't straight, but it was determined.

From there, he dove into the demanding world of old-school medicine: early morning hospital rounds, full office days, late-night follow-ups, and calls to patients after hours. I remember nights when the phone would ring and he'd pick up without hesitation. Sometimes it meant leaving the house; other times it meant simply offering calm reassurance to a worried patient on the other end of the line. To me, as a kid, it seemed ordinary; that's just what Dad did. But as I grew older, I realized the quiet consistency of those moments: the way he carried responsibility without complaint, the way he blended knowledge with compassion.

He paved the path for my brothers and me. All of us pursued medicine — not because he forced us, but because his example made it feel less like a career and more like a calling. We didn't inherit the profession; we inherited the passion.

Now, in my own exam room, I catch glimpses of him in the way I work, in the calm tone I use when I deliver difficult news, in the way I sit down and listen before rushing to a diagnosis, in the steadiness I try to bring to patients who are scared or uncertain. I don't always realize it in the moment, but later I'll think, "That sounded like Dad."

The older I get, the more I understand: My father didn't just teach me about medicine; he taught me about presence. And that, more than anything, is what I try to carry forward.

Now, as a father of three, I understand how hard that balance really is. Each of my kids needs something different. One needs space. One needs time. One needs to be held. I try to divide myself in a way that feels whole to each of them — because more than anything, I want them to feel loved, protected, and seen.

Quieting the Noise

Every day brings a new challenge. Some come from patients, some from administrative headaches. Others come from the unpredictability of life itself. I don't walk into the day assuming I know how it will unfold. Instead, I try to meet it with a steady mind.

That mindset didn't come naturally. For years, I was a chronic overthinker — always forecasting, second-guessing, spiraling. In some ways, that hyperawareness pushed me forward; it kept me sharp, driven, prepared. But it also cost me mental energy, confidence, peace. My mind was crowded with what-ifs, should-haves, and self-doubt. And the truth is, it was exhausting.

Learning to quiet that noise, to stay present for my patients and my children, has been one of the hardest lessons of my life. And one of the most necessary.

That's a hard mindset to carry — especially in a field full of people who seem confident, where patients look to you for certainty and steadiness. For years, I lacked that internal confidence. I felt it, deeply, I just never showed it. I had to learn to quiet the noise and let experience do the talking.

High school, college, medical school, residency — each step shaped who I am. Each one humbled me, challenged me, grounded me more in reality.

I wasn't the top student. I wasn't the star athlete. I went to a small private school about 30 minutes from home. I was a regular kid, trying to figure it all out.

I remember having to give a speech to my entire ninth grade class. I was petrified — sweating, heart racing, mind spinning. That fear didn't mean I wasn't capable; it meant I wasn't prepared for the emotional toll. But I got up there and did it, and strangely, something clicked.

It wasn't that the nerves disappeared — they didn't. But I learned that fear didn't have to disqualify me. I could feel it, carry it with me, and still move forward. That lesson stayed with me. Later, in medicine, I felt it again — the first patient encounter on my own, the first time I had to deliver difficult news, the first time I was trusted to make a decision with real consequences. My heart would race, my mind would spin, but I showed up anyway.

That ninth-grade speech taught me something I've carried ever since: Courage isn't the absence of fear; it's the willingness to act in spite of it.

Now, my whole life is a form of public speaking — walking into exam rooms, meeting strangers, building trust in 10 seconds or less. That same fear is there sometimes. It's quieter now. Familiar. Manageable.

What keeps me grounded isn't some profound mantra; it's the experiences that shaped me. It's my family, my patients, my colleagues. It's the people around me who remind me — intentionally or not — that I'm no better than anyone else — and I never want to be.

I worked hard for what I have. I don't take it for granted. I don't walk through life with assumptions. I try to meet each moment as it is, not as I expect it to be. Over time, I've come to realize I don't have all the answers. I get overwhelmed. I stumble. Yet when I do, I take a breath. I remember my purpose. I return to the people I love.

Being grounded isn't a destination; it's a practice. And like any practice, it requires intention. I lose it, then find it again. I drift, then return. Again and again. That rhythm — the falling and the rising, the losing and the returning — is what keeps me steady in medicine, in writing, in fatherhood, in marriage. Grounded not because life is easy, but because I've learned that presence is the most important place to stand.

The Lessons Parenthood Teaches

I care for many patients who struggle to get pregnant. They try and try — fertility treatments, alternative paths, adoption, surrogacy. The emotional toll is heavy. The journey is long. For so long, I thought having children was simply something that happened. But it isn't always that simple.

I remember sitting with one patient who had endured years of infertility treatments. Appointment after appointment, procedure after procedure, hope rising and falling with every test result. One afternoon, she paused in the middle of our visit and said quietly, "People keep telling me it will happen when it's supposed to. But what if it doesn't?" There was no clinical algorithm for that moment. No guideline or evidence-based pathway that could answer her fear. All I could offer was presence — to listen, to acknowledge the uncertainty, and to understand that for many families, parenthood is not a guarantee but a fragile hope carried forward one day at a time. Moments like that reshaped how I understood the privilege of becoming a parent myself.

Even after conception, the nine months can feel like a lifetime — filled with uncertainty, worry, hope, and fear. Will the baby be okay? Will everything work out?

I never imagined myself as a father of three. Honestly, having just one child felt overwhelming at first. I think that's true for many parents — the first child forces you to learn how to be a parent while simultaneously figuring out who your child is. Why is the baby crying? Is she hungry? Does he need a diaper change? Is she tired? You're left guessing, hoping you're reading the signs correctly, because they can't yet tell you what they need.

I remember one night early on, pacing the hallway with my first child in my arms, convinced I was doing everything wrong. The house was quiet except for the soft rhythm of footsteps across the floor and the steady, uncertain sound of newborn cries. I checked the diaper. Fed him again. Rocked him gently. Nothing seemed to work. I stood there feeling helpless in a way medicine had never prepared me for. There was no differential diagnosis for fatherhood. No attending physician to call. Only instinct, patience, and the quiet realization that sometimes the answer is simply staying present until the moment passes.

By the time our second child arrived, things felt different. Not easier — parenting is never easy — but we had grown. We understood the emotional investment, the patience, the love, and the discipline required to raise a child. We began to understand the delicate balance that makes parenting possible.

And then came our third child. Another girl. She smiles constantly, watching her brother and sister with wide-eyed curiosity, wanting to be just like them. Being a father of two had prepared me to be the best father I could be for her. I learned to slow down. To savor the small moments. I love holding her close. I love watching her light up when she sees her siblings. I love watching all three of them together — laughing, playing, becoming themselves in ways I could never script or predict.

My wife and I have become the strongest team I know. Together, we've built something beautiful.

Cannon shines in swimming and baseball. I remember when he first started — nervous even to compete, unsure if he belonged. Now he's grown into a leader among his peers. He works hard. He supports teammates. He congratulates others whether he wins or loses. He may not always win the race or the game, but he wins in character. And to me, that matters most.

My daughter Cyra is a superstar — sweet and sassy all at once. She loves gymnastics. She adores her brother. And she constantly challenges us as parents. She taught me how to be a true girl dad — how to be patient, how to navigate big emotions, how to lean in instead of pulling away.

She also taught me another important lesson: when you have multiple children, everyone wants attention.

That may be one of the hardest parts of parenting — giving everyone the time, love, and presence they deserve. Not just your children. Your spouse. Your parents. Your friends. Your patients. Yourself.

Parenting isn't only about being present. It's about learning how to balance presence across every role you hold. It is a constant exercise in time, attention, and grace. And every day, I try to get just a little better at it.

Medicine asks for the same thing. Each patient wants to feel heard. Each deserves presence. Just like my children, they arrive with different needs — some seek reassurance, others need answers, and many simply need to know you are truly listening.

Parenting taught me something medicine quietly reinforces every day: being present isn't about dividing yourself perfectly. It's about showing up fully, one person at a time.

The Discipline of Showing Up

But presence is not effortless. It requires energy — emotional, mental, and physical. And over time, I learned that showing up fully for others meant learning how to sustain myself first.

For me, sustaining presence begins when the world is still asleep. I love to move. To sweat. To challenge the version of myself from yesterday. At four in the morning, there's no traffic — just me and the occasional deer crossing an empty road. I pull into the gym. It's silent. Empty. Perfect.

Time disappears there. I forget it's dark outside. By the time I return home, the sky is still black, the house still quiet, and I feel clear-headed, grounded, alive.

Do I want to wake up at four in the morning? Of course not. But I have a wife, three children, a full-time medical practice, and people who depend on me — patients, colleagues, and family. So I carve out time when no one else needs me. Taking care of myself is how I take care of them.

There are mornings when the alarm feels unforgiving — especially after a restless night or a long day before it. On those mornings, the negotiation begins immediately. Stay in bed. Skip today. Start tomorrow. But I've learned that discipline isn't built on convenience. It is built on consistency. And every time I step into the quiet darkness of early morning, I remind myself that showing up for myself is part of showing up for everyone else.

Over time, I've come to look forward to those mornings. Not because they are easy, but because I know how I will feel afterward. That post-workout clarity stays with me throughout the day. It helps me show up fully — for my patients, my team, and most importantly, my family. After work, my time belongs to them. That isn't just a priority. It's a promise.

I chose this life, and I wouldn't trade it for anything. But I've learned you cannot pour from an empty cup. Once the day begins, there is little room for self-reflection. Patients, responsibilities, and decisions fill every hour. So I move early. It clears the mental fog. It centers me. It reminds me that I can carry the weight of other people's stories with care.

That is my responsibility — to be steady, present, and dependable. My patients expect it. My family deserves it.

If you have ever exercised early in the morning, you understand that it is not just physical. It is mental. Emotional. Sometimes even spiritual. That quiet, early-morning discipline carries into every other part of life. Even after nights of poor sleep, I maintain the habit. The discipline becomes stronger than the excuse. The reward always outweighs the effort.

Comfort is always tempting. Sleep in. Skip the workout. Start tomorrow. But comfort rarely builds strength. And strength — physical, mental, emotional — is what carries us through the demands of medicine and life.

Change rarely waits until life becomes easier. It begins when you decide it begins. Not next week. Not when the schedule clears. Now.

You don't grow stronger by thinking about change. You grow stronger by showing up — especially when it feels difficult. The version of yourself you hope to become is waiting on the other side of daily effort.

Exercise grounds me. It sharpens my presence. It reminds me that caring for others begins with caring for myself.

That discipline flows into every part of my life. In medicine, it appears as patience during long clinic days, stamina during difficult conversations, and humility in the face of constant learning. In marriage, it appears in small daily choices — conversations after exhausting days, forgiveness after misunderstandings, and the quiet decision to keep choosing each other again and again.

The gym was never about building muscle. It was about building mindset. It was about practicing presence in quiet hours so I could live it out when the world demanded it.

Medicine, marriage, and fatherhood all require the same thing: consistency. Not perfection — persistence. Not ease — endurance.

And that is the life I have built. One early morning, one patient encounter, one family moment at a time.

The Essence of Role Models

Growing up, I believed something simple but powerful: to be the best, you have to learn from the best. For me, that meant my parents.

My father was a gastroenterologist who practiced both internal medicine and GI. My mother was the steady presence who made everything possible. My dad showed up for his patients every day, and my mom showed up for us. Together, they formed the foundation that shaped who I am — as a doctor, a father, and a person.

Their lives were a model of consistency, of commitment. My dad's staff loved him. His patients trusted him. And at home, we trusted our mom the same way. She never missed a beat. She never made us feel like an inconvenience, no matter how early the morning or how packed the day.

They modeled kindness, consistency, and quiet strength. The lesson they lived by was simple: Take care of people the way you'd take care of your family. And that's what I carry into my office every day.

Some of my strongest memories aren't of hospital corridors or white coats — they're of hockey rinks at six in the morning, in the middle of a Boston winter. My dad, freezing in the stands but smiling. Afterward, we'd go to Perfecto's for a bagel and coffee — our little ritual. And while we were doing that, my mom was at home waking up my siblings, getting everyone moving, making sure the day stayed on track.

Those little routines were never little. They were the rhythm of our lives. They were how love showed up.

They taught us what it means to work hard, to stay kind, and to be dependable. My dad smiled no matter how long the day. My mom never let us see how tired she must have been. She kept going. He kept going. And they kept showing up — not for recognition, but because that's who they were.

A train doesn't run with only a conductor; you also need an engineer. In our family, my father may have steered the professional direction, but my mother kept everything moving. She made the system work. She built the structure and the soul of our home. Yet, there was no hierarchy. Just a true partnership — steady, strong, and aligned. They raised four kids with purpose, with joy, and with endless support. I always knew I could count on them — win or lose, pass or fail. As I found my own path in medicine, they were always there. Not pushing. Just believing, trusting, guiding.

They never gave long lectures. They didn't need to. Their actions were louder. I learned how to care, how to show up, and how to lead from watching them live their lives. I learned that love and work can coexist. That you can be tired and still be present. That true strength is quiet, constant, and unwavering.

They taught me that success isn't measured by degrees or titles; it's measured in people, in impact, in presence — the act of being wholly there.

I smile when I walk into my office because I carry their example with me. I treat each patient like family. I show up for my kids like they did for me. For when you learn from the best — when you're raised by the best — you carry that forward.

The moral of this story is simple: Never forget where you came from. Make the most of the opportunities given to you. That's what my parents did, and that's what I strive to do every day.

The Circle of Trust

I've never needed to be the center of attention. I've never craved the spotlight or chased social circles to be seen. I'm not wired that way. I've always been more comfortable behind the scenes — quietly doing the work, showing up for others, staying grounded in what matters. What I have come to understand — through experience, observation, and some hard truths — is that life is better, healthier, and more meaningful when you keep a tight circle.

Your parents, your kids, a few close friends, a handful of colleagues — these are the people who show up not just when it's easy, but also when it's hard. They are the ones who support your choices not blindly, but with grace. They'll cheer you on, but they'll also hold you accountable. They want the best for you, even when it means telling you something you don't want to hear. That's real love. That's trust. That's loyalty. I have come to understand that loyalty is a quiet, powerful force. It's not loud, it's not flashy, it's not the person tagging you in a post or clapping the loudest at your wins. It's the person who shows up when there's nothing to gain. The one who doesn't tolerate your lowest moments but stays, listens, and helps you get through them.

In my own life, I've been fortunate to have people I can trust. Farah — my anchor and confidant — has stood beside me through seasons of doubt, long nights, and professional pivots. My kids remind me daily of what matters. They don't care about titles or accolades; they care about presence, and that's what grounds me.

The people in my circle of trust have become my sounding boards, my day-to-day sanity, my friends. We've shared stories, frustrations, small victories. We've covered for each other when the day gets overwhelming and checked in even when no one asked us to. That's not part of a job description; that's part of being human.

I've also been let down. I've trusted people who didn't deserve it. I've confided in people who turned around and used it for gossip or leverage. I've seen people act like allies when the cameras are on, only to disappear the moment they're no longer in the spotlight. Those moments sting, but they also teach. They remind you who belongs in your circle — and who doesn't.

Over time, I've come to understand that not everyone deserves access to your life. Just because someone wants your time, your energy, your attention, that doesn't mean they've earned it. Not everyone who smiles in your face is cheering for you. Some are waiting for their chance to benefit from your success or quietly hoping you stumble.

I don't say that with cynicism. I say it with clarity, with peace. Because the truth is this: Fewer, deeper relationships are worth far more than a crowd of surface-level ones. Showing up fully for a handful of people matters more than stretching yourself thin trying to please everyone. Being known isn't nearly as important as being understood.

So I protect my circle. I value the people who value me. I give my energy to those who pour theirs into me. That's not selfish — it's sustainable.

If you've found your people, hold onto them. Cherish them. Nurture those relationships. If you haven't, keep looking. Be open. Be kind. Be the kind of friend you wish you had. There are good people out there — people who will lift you up, not tear you down. People who will stand beside you even when there's nothing in it for them.

For loyalty is rare. Real friendship is rare. And when you find it, you protect it. Keep your circle tight. Make it real. Make it honest.

The world doesn't need more noise — it needs more genuine, grounded, loyal connection.

In the end, it always comes back to the people: the mentors who guided me when I felt lost, the friends who stood beside me in difficult moments, the family who supported my dreams and believed in my potential.

They are the reason I can do this work. This was never just my story — it's ours.

The Ubiquity of Being a Care Giver

This profession isn't something you clock out of; it lingers, waiting, ready to surface when you least expect it. It happened one night in Orlando, before a family cruise, and I will never forget it.

The night before our cruise, we decided to spend the evening at Disney Springs. Farah and I thought it would be fun for the kids — something low-key before we boarded the ship the next morning. Neon lights glowed on the water. Families in vacation T-shirts milled about, laughter echoing from every direction. We chose the House of Blues for dinner.

It was supposed to be a normal night. We sat at our table — my wife, our two kids at the time, and my in-laws — settling into the familiar rhythm of dining out. The kids squabbled over who got which seat, my in-laws looked over the menu, and we ordered drinks and an appetizer. We were ready to begin what felt like a well-deserved week of escape.

And then I heard it. A voice from directly behind me. Trembling, uneven, sharp with panic.

"Help me, please."

I froze for a split second, and then instinct took over. I turned in my chair and saw an older gentleman seated at the table behind ours. He was upright, but barely. His head sagged forward, his body slack against the chair. His chest heaved in shallow gasps, his eyes distant, unfocused. He wasn't responding. He wasn't alert. He was sitting there, actively dying.

There was no time to think, only to move. As I shot out of my seat, his daughter, sitting beside him, reached for her father, her face stricken with disbelief. A few bystanders moved toward us. As gently but as quickly as we could, we lowered him onto the restaurant floor amid the clatter of plates and the rising murmur of onlookers.

I ripped open his shirt, laid a hand on his chest, and searched for a pulse. Nothing. "Start compressions," I said. And we did.

It's strange how the world shrinks in a moment like that. Just seconds earlier, I'd been settling in for dinner. Now the only reality was a man's silent chest beneath my hands, the rhythm of compression, the fragile line between life and death.

The daughter cried out for her father, clutching his arm as strangers pressed into service beside me. A busboy, in his apron, sprinted over, kneeling next to us. Another guest had already called 911. Someone ran to retrieve an AED. We were a team now, strangers woven together by urgency, united by the singular goal of giving this man another chance at life.

The AED arrived. The pads were placed, sticky against his bare chest. "Analyzing rhythm," the machine intoned in its cold, mechanical voice. Shock advised.

Everyone stood back. Clear. His body jerked as the current coursed through him. Still no pulse.

Compressions resumed. Rhythmical, relentless. I could hear the daughter sobbing, pleading, "Come back, Dad, come back."

The AED reanalyzed. Again: Shock advised. Clear. Another jolt.

This time, something changed. His chest rose. A gasp. His face regained color. A flutter at his neck — a pulse. Breath. Life.

I sat back on my heels, sweating, trembling, hardly able to believe what I was seeing. He was awake. He was breathing normally. His pulse was back. By the time EMS arrived minutes later, he was stable enough to be transferred. They placed him on a stretcher, monitors beeping, oxygen flowing, and rolled him out of the restaurant. His daughter bent over him, crying, now with relief instead of despair. Before she left, she hugged me — wordless, desperate, grateful — and then she was gone.

Just like that, the moment passed. The clatter of dishes resumed. Servers shuffled back into motion. The world continued on, as if nothing had happened. But everything had changed.

Later that night, in the hotel room, the kids couldn't stop mimicking the motion of chest compressions, pressing down on their pillows, giggling nervously, trying to process it. "Like this, Daddy?" they asked, pushing rhythmically, mimicking the life-saving motion.

That night, I couldn't sleep. The scene replayed in my mind over and over: the gasping, the silence, the compressions, the shocks. But what stayed with me even more was not the man on the floor — it was my kids, seated behind me the entire time, watching.

They had seen everything. They saw their dad spring up from the table and drop to the floor. They saw strangers rally together to try to bring a man back to life. They saw me kneeling, sweat dripping, counting compressions, barking for people to stand clear. They saw the shocks, the jolts, the color return, the breath come back. They saw a man die — and then live again.

They brought it up the next day, and the day after that. And still, every now and then, they mention the man at Disney Springs, the one who collapsed at the table next to us and came back.

It shook me more than I expected. Because in that moment, my kids didn't see Dad; they saw the doctor.

At work, people know me as a physician. But at home, none of that matters. To my kids, I'm the one who tucks them in at night, who drives them to swim meets, who nags them about brushing their teeth. They don't see the diplomas on the wall or the long hours behind the white coat. They just see Dad. And in the end, that's the title I hold most dearly — the one that will never change, no matter what else does. And that's how I want it to be.

But that night, they witnessed something different. They saw that the person who cuts the turkey at Thanksgiving, who reads them bedtime stories, who helps with homework, is also someone who carries knowledge and responsibility into the world. Someone who, when the call comes, doesn't hesitate. Someone who can take part in saving a life.

It was a collision of identities — Dad and Doctor — laid bare in front of them. And in that moment, the two could no longer be separated. It was proof that what I do matters, proof that their father is more than the man who sits at the dinner table, proof that the white coat, even when not worn, is never set aside.

I hope they remember it not with fear, but with a sense of wonder. Not because their dad is a doctor, but because in moments of crisis, ordinary people can rise to do extraordinary things. That night at Disney Springs, they saw humanity at its best.

The truth is, the heroes of that night were not me; they were the daughter who never left her father's side, the busboy who sprinted to help, the strangers who didn't turn away — the ones who, despite fear and inexperience, joined hands in an impossible moment.

The coat is not who I am; it is what I carry into the world. And they saw me not as Dad, but as both.

Reclaiming Humanity

How do we reclaim peace, purpose, and humanity in medicine?

In the end, the practice of medicine is really the practice of being human. And to reclaim that humanity is to remember that we are more than what we fear, and far more than what we fix.

We worry about failing. We worry about succeeding. We worry about how we're perceived, what might go wrong, and how we'll fix things that haven't even broken. Worry can be debilitating — even paralyzing. It creeps into every corner of our lives. It clouds judgment, stalls progress, and robs us of peace. It convinces us not to try, not to risk, not to hope. Worry becomes a full-time job.

I know this truth too well. For years, I worried my way through medicine. I worried about making mistakes, about disappointing a patient, about ordering the wrong test. I worried about being liked, about being respected, about being "good enough." The list was endless, and the weight was crushing. Most of what I feared never happened. Regardless, I paid the price — physically, emotionally, spiritually.

The problem isn't the thought — it's the lens we apply to it. Worry warps that lens. It distorts reality, exaggerates fear, and turns the unknown into a threat. This is magnified in medicine. Patients worry. We worry. A slight abnormality or a minor lab result becomes a catastrophe in our minds, and then we spiral.

Chest pain? The first thought is almost always heart attack. Yet in reality, more often it's anxiety, acid reflux, or a strained muscle. Belly pain? A Google search spits out appendicitis, gallstones, cancer. But more often, it's just something you ate. Maybe bad shrimp or one too many tacos.

This isn't to say symptoms don't deserve attention — they do. But the issue is perspective. And in medicine, perspective is often the first thing we lose.

Most people don't live in the complexity of the human body. To them, every unknown feels like a crisis. Every symptom feels like danger. Every test result becomes a rabbit hole of fear. And worry doesn't stop there. It builds on itself. One fear piles onto the next until we assume the worst. That's what sends us spiraling into despair, into sadness, into exhaustion. A hamster wheel we can't seem to step off. By the time reality settles in and the worst-case scenario never comes to pass, we're left depleted, wondering if all that worry was worth it.

Perspective doesn't eliminate uncertainty; it gives us space to breathe, to think clearly, to be present with what is instead of what might be.

As physicians, we're called to do more than diagnose and treat. We're called to help people navigate their fear, to offer calm in the chaos, to remind them that not every "what if" is a catastrophe waiting to unfold. Without that anchor, the "what ifs" will keep winning and worry will keep writing the story.

But fear doesn't only whisper through worst-case scenarios; sometimes its loudest voice is silence. It shows up in the questions we never ask, the risks we never take, the words we keep inside.

And that's the deeper heartbreak: The hardest sound isn't "no." What cuts deeper is the silence that accompanies the regret of never trying. In medicine, as in life, it is often the questions unasked, the conversations avoided, the risks left untaken that leave the heaviest weight.

I've seen it firsthand: Patients who don't speak up because they're afraid of looking foolish. Students who don't raise their hands because they fear being wrong. Colleagues who don't ask for help because they don't want to seem weak. And in my own life, I've carried those silences too — the questions unasked, the risks not taken, the words I held back.

"No" is definitive, but it's also clarifying. It closes one door while leaving space to find another. Silence, on the other hand, lingers. It haunts. It leaves us wondering forever what might have been.

If someone says no? That's fine. You tried. You found the courage to face the unknown. You overcame the cliffhanger of doubt, and that alone is something to be proud of.

The first step is asking. The second step is handling the response. But don't get stuck on step two before you've even taken step one.

What's been on your mind? What have you been holding back? What's the question you're too afraid to ask? Maybe it's time to stop being so stoic, to stop fearing rejection, to accept defeat when it comes and move forward. Because "no" isn't the end; it's part of the process.

There have been so many moments in my life when I wanted something deeply: an outpatient clinical rotation, a specific role, a better office. And yes, sometimes I hesitated, afraid of seeming entitled, afraid of hearing "no," afraid I'd feel small or inadequate.

Yet over time, I've learned to ask anyway, because the worst they can say is "no." Yes, "no" stings and makes you question your worth. Yet, here's the twist: "No" is clarity. It stops the spiral of overthinking and gives you direction. Figure out what needs to change, and go after it again.

Almost every meaningful step I've taken in life began with a question. Even as a young, nervous student, I asked — sometimes with a shaky voice. I didn't want to look weak; I didn't want to fail. I feared that hearing "no" might break me. Now, I hear it all the time. And I'm sure I'll hear it again.

Am I discouraged? No. I'm energized. Rejection doesn't mean you're unworthy; it means you're still in the arena, you're trying.

So when you hear "no," don't stop. Ask yourself: Why did they say no? What can I improve? Do I need more experience? More confidence? Is it my résumé? My pitch? My timing?

"No" can be the beginning of something greater. It can lead you to something even better than you expected. Sometimes, "no" isn't failure; it's the spark of something fresh, something bold, something that could change your life.

If you don't ask, regret may creep in.

Living Without Regret

I haven't lived a flawless life — far from it. Like anyone who's lived fully, I've made decisions I wouldn't necessarily make again. I've stumbled, hesitated, chosen unwisely, spoken too soon — or too late. I've doubted myself. But I've never looked back on those moments with the word "regret" stamped across them.

Regret, to me, feels static. It's a pause in the story, a freeze-frame of failure that refuses to let the reel keep playing. I've always believed life is about motion — learning, adapting, growing. Even when we falter, we're moving forward, evolving. Regret, by contrast, feels like emotional quicksand.

In medicine, the moments that tempt regret are countless. You can make all the right decisions, follow the guidelines to the letter, and things can still go wrong. That's the nature of the work. That's the weight of it.

Sometimes a diagnosis hides in plain sight, with symptoms so subtle they're easy to overlook. Sometimes a test is delayed, and by the time results come back, the patient's condition has already shifted. Sometimes reassurance is given in good faith — only for the story to change in ways no one could have predicted.

These are not failures of effort or intent; they are the humbling realities of a profession where uncertainty is always part of the equation.

And yet, regret doesn't serve us. Instead, we return to these moments like students. We review the notes. We ask questions. We sharpen our eyes for the next time. That's the quiet contract physicians sign: to keep learning from patients, even when, and especially when, the lessons are hard to swallow.

Regret is easy to fall into, but it rarely serves us. It disguises itself as responsibility, but in truth, it's often self-punishment in a lab coat.

When I think back on my life — on the long, winding path that carried me through medical school, residency, attendinghood, and now leadership — I don't see a straight line. I see detours. I see recalibrations. I see dozens of decisions that, at the time, felt either arbitrary or urgent and only later revealed their meaning.

Life doesn't demand perfection; it demands persistence. Not regret, but reflection. Not paralysis, but progress. It taught me to work harder. It taught me humility. It taught me that your worth is not defined by the stamp on your diploma, but by the depth of your care.

I didn't go to the "right" medical school — at least not according to the standards whispered in conference rooms or printed in rankings. I took a route that many looked down on. And yet, that choice shaped me more than any "perfect" path could have. Had I followed someone else's definition of prestige, I wouldn't be where I am today. I might not even be a doctor. And I certainly wouldn't be the doctor I am now.

I've listened to classmates and colleagues second-guess themselves: Should I have taken that job? Chosen another specialty? Gone to that school? Married that person? Moved to that city? Beneath all those questions lies the same ache — the belief that if only we had chosen differently, we might have unlocked a flawless version of life. But that version doesn't exist. There is no alternate life waiting for us. There is only this one, and it deserves our full attention.

We're taught to aim high, to strive for excellence, to correct our errors. But somewhere along the way, that drive can get tangled up in shame. We stop seeing our past as the foundation of who we are and start seeing it as a series of missteps. That's when regret creeps in.

And here's the irony: Regret feels like reflection. It poses as insight. But it doesn't teach — it punishes. It doesn't propel — it stalls. It replaces action with rumination.

Reflection without regret is more powerful. It allows me to look back on my past self not with judgment, but with compassion. That young doctor was doing the best he could with what he knew. He was showing up, asking questions, staying late, and learning fast. He didn't always get it right, but he kept going and he grew.

That's what matters.

Even outside of medicine, this philosophy holds. We miss calls. We say the wrong thing. We put off plans, skip important conversations, choose work over rest or rest over work. We can't rewind the tape, but we can carry the lesson forward.

Would I do everything the same? No. Do I regret it? Still no. Because each misstep made me more intentional. Each hard moment gave me a new lens. Each wrong turn taught me how to find my way back.

Regret, to me, is a closed door. Learning is a hallway with light on both ends.

That doesn't mean I move through life without accountability. It means I practice accountability with grace. I ask: What did I miss? What can I do better next time? What does this teach me about who I'm becoming?

When my patients struggle with their own pasts — regretting that they didn't come in sooner, that they didn't take better care of themselves, that they didn't listen to the signs their bodies were trying to send — I remind them that the most important decision is the one you make now. You're here. You're engaged. You're trying. That counts. That's everything.

We are not the sum of our regrets. We are the product of our response to them.

So no, I don't believe in regrets. I believe in adaptation. I believe in perspective. I believe in the version of me that existed yesterday, and the version that will exist tomorrow. I trust them both. For they are the same person — trying, learning, becoming.

Welcome to My World

Sometimes I look out the window of my office and can't believe this is real. I have an office. It's mine — not rented, not borrowed. Inside sits a desk that's both cluttered and meaningful, patient charts stacked with stories, and a chair that witnesses more emotion in a week than some people see in a year. To some, it might look like nothing more than a room with a window. But to me, it's a symbol, a milestone, a quiet reminder of how far I've come.

There was a time, not so long ago, when I never imagined this would be my life. I never thought I'd make it into medical school. I never thought I'd survive the relentless pace once I got there. I never thought I'd match into residency, let alone pass boards that felt insurmountable at the time. I never thought I'd be someone a patient would call "my doctor."

There were no shortcuts. No guarantees. No promises. Just work. Just grit. And just enough belief in myself.

The office is proof of that. But it's more than proof — it's a responsibility. The walls don't just hold my achievements; they hold the trust of every patient who walks through the door. They carry the weight of quiet confessions, hard questions, unexpected tears, and moments of relief.

I remember one afternoon when a longtime patient sat across from me, tears spilling down her face as she told me her husband had died the week before. She wasn't there for labs or prescriptions — she was there because she didn't know where else to go. She wanted someone who knew her story, who would sit in silence with her grief.

I didn't offer a diagnosis or a treatment plan. I simply bore witness. When she finally stood to leave, she squeezed my hand and said, "Thank you for seeing me — not just as a patient, but as a person."

When I look around my office, I don't just see charts or medical degrees. I see a space that holds people's stories — their laughter, their fears, their tears. It's not the walls that matter; it's what they've contained. That is the real symbol of how far I've come.

Every chart on my desk is a story in progress. Every seat filled in front of me is a life unfolding in real time. And every day, I'm reminded that this space isn't just about me; it's about the people who believe enough in me to let me be part of their story.

And when I think about the long, winding road that led here — the detours, the doubts, the moments that felt like failures — I don't see regrets. I see the lessons that shaped me. I see persistence. I see the grit that turned uncertainty into purpose.

Because the office isn't the end of the story; it's a checkpoint, a reminder that perfection was never the goal — persistence was, growth was. And those are what brought me here.

Still, I didn't get here alone; I also had people who stood beside me during my lowest moments. People who guided me when I was unsure of what came next. Mentors who challenged me — not with sugarcoated words, but with honesty. Friends who believed in me even when I couldn't. Family members who reminded me that my worth was never tied to test scores or titles. I'm deeply grateful for all of them.

I've come to understand that success isn't a solo sport. Even the smallest victory carries the fingerprints of others — the ones who paved the way, who pushed me forward, who whispered "Keep going" when I wasn't sure I could. That's why I hold so tightly to gratitude. It keeps me grounded, human.

And on the days when the pressure mounts — when the inbox overflows, the EMR drags, and I feel pulled in every direction — I take a breath and remind myself: This is a privilege. I get to do this.

I get to be part of people's lives in a way few others can. I get to listen to their stories, interpret their pain, help them carry their fears. I get to be trusted — not with symptoms, but with secrets. Not with diagnoses, but with hope.

A patient walks into my office and tells me about their mother's declining memory. Or their chest pain. Or the loss they haven't spoken to anyone about. And they tell me. Me. That's not routine. That's sacred.

I don't take it lightly that someone chooses to sit across from me and unravel what's been tightly wound inside them. Whether it's a quiet "I'm not okay" or a brave "Can I tell you something I've never told anyone before?" — these moments matter. These moments are why I chose medicine in the first place.

So yes, I have an office. I have a full panel, a leadership role, and a calendar that rarely has white space. Yet none of that means anything without the gratitude that fuels it all.

The sleepless nights in med school. The lonely rotations far from home. The call shifts when I doubted everything. The whispered "what if I'm not good enough" moments that tried to define me. Those became teachers. They turned hardship into growth, failure into resilience, fear into focus.

I'm thankful to be here.

Thankful to be alive.

Thankful for a family who sees me as more than a doctor.

Thankful for colleagues who lift me up when I feel the weight of this profession.

Thankful for patients who, unknowingly, teach me more about life than any textbook ever could.

I'm thankful for the chance to keep learning, evolving, becoming.

This journey is far from over — and I welcome that. I'll continue forward with open hands and a steady heart. I'll face new challenges. I'll walk into the unknown, not with fear, but with a quiet confidence built on years of climbing uphill.

Because if there's one thing I've come to understand, it's this: The road doesn't get easier; you get better at walking it.

And through it all, I won't forget who I am. I won't forget where I came from. I won't forget the sacrifices, the support, the slow build that got me here. I won't forget the voices that said "yes" when others said "maybe." The people who opened doors I never knew existed. The ones who didn't give me handouts — but gave me a chance.

That's why I give back now. That's why I invest in others. Because someone once did that for me. I live by a simple philosophy: If you help me, I'll help you.

Whether it's mentoring a young physician, supporting a colleague, or listening a little longer to a patient who needs to be heard — I pay it forward.

I choose to lead with compassion.

To practice with humility.

To live with intention.

I choose to keep going.

To keep saying thank you — not only with words, but with how I show up in the world.

Because this life — the one I never thought I'd have — is a gift.

And every time I look out that window, I remember: I'm exactly where I'm meant to be.

EPILOGUE

This brings the journey full circle: Medicine has never been about absolutes, but about persistence, compassion, and the quiet, stubborn courage to keep showing up. In the end, what endures is not certainty, but courage itself.

BECAUSE MEDICINE, AT ITS CORE, is about presence and humanity.

For years, I thought I knew what success looked like: overbooked days, inboxes overflowing, lunches skipped, breathing shallow between patients. But I have come to understand that being busy is not the same as being fulfilled. Patients do not long for flawless doctors; they long to be seen.

Somewhere along the way, medicine shifted. We navigate portals. We spend more time documenting care than delivering it. In the name of efficiency, we risk forgetting why most of us entered this profession in the first place: to care, to heal, to connect.

I remember nights finishing charts long after my last patient had gone, the clinic dark except for the glow of the computer screen. My eyes blurred from endless clicks. I wondered how many minutes I had spent documenting instead of listening. The paradox of modern medicine is that the more data we capture, the more story we risk losing. And yet, behind every lab, every inbox message, every scanned report is a person. That is the truth I refuse to let the system erase.

I did not go to medical school to become a data-entry specialist. I went to learn how to listen. How to sit with someone who is scared. How to explain what no one else has taken the time to explain. How to be there, not just as a physician, but as a steady presence in someone's most vulnerable moments.

Of course, medicine has always demanded that we be right. Lives depend on accuracy, and science is our compass. But I have come to understand that correctness alone is not enough. A diagnosis delivered without compassion is incomplete. A treatment plan explained without empathy falls short. To heal fully, we must be both right and present.

And yet, as doctors, we are rarely granted that same grace. We are expected to absorb grief, anger, and uncertainty and keep going. To never show weakness. To never need help. But we are not immune to the weight of it all.

Some nights, I sat in the driveway, the engine idling, dashboard lights casting a tired glow across my hands as I gathered myself before walking inside. Through the windows I could hear life continuing — children laughing, toys scattered across the floor, the smell of dinner lingering. Crossing that threshold meant shifting from doctor to dad, from carrying loss to carrying love.

Cannon's glove snapping with each pitch. Cyra's laughter sharp and unrestrained. Camille's syrup-sticky fingers clutching mine. Those were the sounds that reminded me resilience is not about shutting out the grief, but about allowing joy to coexist with it.

I have come to understand that boundaries are not selfish; they are survival. That we do not have to choose between being good doctors and whole people. That strength can be found in vulnerability, and power in admitting that this is hard.

Medicine is not broken because doctors do not care. It is strained because we care so deeply with so few outlets to carry the weight. We need a system that supports our humanity, not one that suppresses it.

Because in the end, patients do not want perfection. They want presence. They want to be seen, heard, and understood, not by an algorithm, but by a person. And that starts with letting doctors be people, too.

My story is not unique. Countless others walk this same road, grappling with uncertainty, chasing purpose, carrying the weight of medicine. This book has been my attempt to give voice to that shared reality, to capture what it feels like to live inside the white coat, with all its doubts and resilience, quiet victories and stinging failures, the balance between science and soul.

What endures is not certainty, but connection. Not perfection, but persistence. Not data, but the human story.

And so this is where my story leaves off, not with an ending, but with a beginning still unfolding. Not with perfection, but with presence. Not with certainty, but with honesty.

Because the practice of medicine, at its core,
is not only about being right.
It is about being present.
It is about staying human.
And that is where I choose to remain.

www.ingramcontent.com/pod-product-compliance
Lightning Source LLC
Chambersburg PA
CBHW071445230926
51846CB00001B/344
* 9 7 8 1 9 6 0 7 6 2 5 5 9 *